DIETS, MALNUTRITION, AND DISEASE

DIETS, MALNUTRITION, AND DISEASE

The Indian Experience

edited by
RAGHAV GAIHA
RAGHBENDRA JHA
VANI S. KULKARNI

OXFORD
UNIVERSITY PRESS

OXFORD
UNIVERSITY PRESS

Oxford University Press is a department of the University of Oxford.
It furthers the University's objective of excellence in research, scholarship,
and education by publishing worldwide. Oxford is a registered trademark of
Oxford University Press in the UK and in certain other countries

Published in India by
Oxford University Press
YMCA Library Building, 1 Jai Singh Road, New Delhi 110 001, India

First Edition published in 2014

ISBN-13: 978-0-19-809921-5
ISBN-10: 0-19-809921-5

Typeset in Bembo Std 10.5/13
by SPEX Infotech, Puducherry, India 605 005
Printed in India at Rakmo Press, New Delhi 110 020

Raghav Gaiha...

to Inder, a close friend who was snatched away by the cruel hand of fate. His lifelong devotion and commitment to the cause of better health for disadvantaged women were exemplary, matched only by his personal generosity

Raghbendra Jha...

to Alka and Abhay

Vani S. Kulkarni...

to her late father—a loving father and a brilliant scholar—for making her academic pursuits so meaningful and rewarding

Contents

Tables and Figures

TABLES

FIGURES

Foreword

C. Peter Timmer*

India has presented an enigma to several generations of development specialists. The 'Hindu rate of growth' of 2 per cent per year per capita, when East and Southeast Asia exceeded 5 per cent, was an early issue. The surprisingly rapid response to economic liberalization in the 1990s resolved that issue but raised another; in an increasingly globalized and competitive world, would India's economic policies be adequate to meet the new challenge from China? And from the perspective of the second decade of the new millennium, another important puzzle emerged: why is rapid economic growth not transforming the diets and health of the poor, especially in rural areas?

This volume edited by Raghav Gaiha, Raghbendra Jha, and Vani S. Kulkarni seeks to answer the third question directly, within the broader context of the evolution of India's economy and policy arena. The editors, three of the most respected academics working on Indian food policy and poverty dynamics, bring a breadth of analytical techniques to rich data sets, and then place their analysis in the context of India's perplexing political economy. Each chapter tackles a specific aspect of the issue, and each rewards careful study and thought.

* C. Peter Timmer is the Cabot Professor of Development Studies, Emeritus, Harvard University, and Adjunct Professor, Crawford School of Public Policy, Australian National University. He can be reached at ptimmer63@gmail.com.

Befitting its large role in the developing world, India's approaches to solving these problems have attracted very high-profile attention. In particular, a careful comparative study of contrasting approaches to their food and agricultural sectors in India and China, coordinated by International Food Policy Research Institute (IFPRI), sheds empirical and policy light on many of the issues in this volume (Gulati and Fan 2007). My review in *Science* made the following observations about the competition between China and India, and their contrasting experiences with food and agriculture:

> The volume seeks to understand the foundations of the Chinese and Indian growth successes and finds them, not surprisingly, in efforts in both countries to revitalize their rural economies. Such revitalization was essential, the various authors argue, if the massive and impoverished populations in each country were to have any hope of higher living standards, including enough food to eat. The spectre of hunger was a basic driver of reform policy in both China and India.
>
> Three main themes drive the story of rural reforms in China and India. First, China started well behind India in 1950 in terms of poverty, institutional infrastructure, and mechanisms of governance. Both countries struggled for 30 years to find a path to inclusive modernization. But to most observers' surprise, China found the path sooner, exploited it faster, and has roared past India in nearly all indicators of economic success. Only India's democratic form of governance (flawed as it is) holds promise for convergence in the future.
>
> Second, and no doubt controversially, China's 'initial conditions' laid down during the Maoist era are now seen to provide substantial advantages in managing rapid, inclusive growth. Greater gender equality, investments in rural human and physical capital, even the capacity to control policy from the centre, now make the Maoist experiment with collectivization and rigid central planning seem not the disaster it appeared to be in the late 1970s.
>
> Third, details matter. They matter at both a strategic level and at the level of commodity-specific, region-specific approaches to agricultural development. Here, the volume is rich in specificity about contrasts in China's and India's approaches to the 'big' rural reform issues: trade policy (China opted early on for a much more open approach); poverty alleviation (China opted for rapid growth in rural areas, whereas India retained a state-provided safety net that became increasingly cumbersome and expensive); rural non-farm economy (India is only

> now beginning to facilitate the natural vibrancy of rural entrepreneurs investing to service their agricultural neighbours).
>
> Looking forward, it is hard to miss the pessimism of the Indian authors as they look at their country's rural reforms and progress compared with China's. The chapter by V.S. Vyas, the 'dean' of agricultural economists in India, is titled 'Market Reforms in Indian Agriculture: One Step Forward and Two Steps Back'. And here is the not-so-hidden agenda of the volume: the final sentence of the Acknowledgments says, 'We are most grateful to Indian Prime Minister Manmohan Singh, the architect of economic reforms in India, who inaugurated the first conference in New Delhi and is still keen to know what each country can learn from the other' (p. xxii). Competition works in powerful ways, even in the world of political economy (Timmer 2008: 642).

A much sharper focus on the deep health and education problems facing India comes from two of its best-known analysts (Sen and Dréze 2013). A review of the Sen and Dréze volume in *The Economist* highlights the issues:

> As a conundrum it could hardly be bigger. Six decades of laudably fair elections, a free press, rule of law, and much else should have delivered rulers who are responsive to the ruled. India's development record, however, is worse than poor. It is host to some of the world's worst failures in health and education. If democracy works, why are so many Indian lives still so wretched?
>
> Social indicators leave that in no doubt. A massive blackout last summer (2012) caught global attention, yet 400 million Indians had (and still have) no electricity. Sanitation and public hygiene are awful, especially in the north: half of all Indians still defecate in the open, resulting in many deaths from diarrhoea and encephalitis. Polio may be gone, but immunization rates for most diseases are lower than in sub-Saharan Africa. Twice as many Indian children (43 per cent) as African ones go hungry.
>
> Many adults, especially women, are also undernourished, even as obesity and diabetes spread among wealthier Indians. Despite gains, extreme poverty is rife and death in childbirth is all too common. Prejudice kills on an immense scale: as many as 600,000 foetuses are aborted each year because they are female. Compared even with its poorer neighbours, Bangladesh and Nepal, India's social record is unusually grim. (*The Economist* 2013: 74)

Against this record, Gaiha, Jha, and Kulkarni offer documentation of the problems as well as insights into solutions. Three basic forces seem to be driving most of their empirical investigations, with direct consequences for how policies might be brought to bear in bringing about improvements. The authors are understandably cautious in claiming to have understood these problems well enough to offer full-blown policy recommendations. In fact, evidence-based policy formulation tends to be incremental and learns as it goes (Timmer *et al.* 1983).

First, incomes at the household level are critical for nearly all of the problems under analysis: demand for nutrients, the dietary transition from reliance on starchy staples to a much more diversified diet, the measurement of malnutrition, the prevalence of poverty traps in rural areas and of child malnutrition, the increasing incidence of non-communicable diseases and health problems of the aeging and affluent, even the prevalence of leakages from targeted programmes to subsidize food intake or guarantee work opportunities. Perhaps it is not surprising that even sophisticated econometric techniques do not displace incomes as the leading driver of nutritional outcomes. Choice matters and higher incomes provide greater freedom of choice. If the reader takes only one message away from this volume, it is the critical importance of continuing the drive to increase per capita incomes in India, not just on average, but among the poor, where it really matters.

Second, absolute and relative prices matter to food consumption and to nutritional outcomes. For someone who wrote a book on 'getting prices right' more than a quarter of a century ago (Timmer 1986), the continued relevance and significant impact of food prices is satisfying, but not surprising. After all, market economies depend on price formation to send signals to producers and consumers about what to grow and what to eat. If these signals are distorted or ignored, the whole market paradigm falls apart. But we have nothing to replace it, certainly not state planning of crop production and rationing of consumption goods. We need prices to work.

Finally, incomes and prices do not come even close to being the whole story in explaining India's perplexing patterns of dietary choices, malnutrition, and disease. Many other variables are at play and the authors are good at teasing them out, even when measurement is difficult—how can individual nutritional requirements be observed, for example? Still, there are powerful, and easily measurable, forces at work. Perhaps the most critical and visible force is gender. From my work in Indonesia, especially with Steve Block, I am easily persuaded that the quality of home care for children, in particular their nutrient intake and healthcare, is highly conditioned by the 'empowerment' of the mother (the authors' term). In turn, this role of women is characterized by a multitude of cultural factors (which economists often take as fixed), but in reality the woman's role in the household can often be enhanced, quite significantly, by educational opportunities and access to family planning services.

Knowledge of good nutritional practices is not hard-wired; it seems to be acquired mostly by observational learning. But we now know, for sure, that it can be taught in school with significant improvements in children's nutritional status as a result (Webb and Block 2004). Any society that cares about the welfare of its children will be working hard to guarantee that women attend school and learn about health and nutrition while they are there.

The bleak status of children's nutritional standing, especially in rural India, has its parallels in China as well. A team from Stanford University working with Chinese scientists has documented the depth of malnutrition among school-age children in rural China and has started a campaign to mobilize additional resources and policy attention from the government. Early malnutrition can cause severe cognitive impairment, and permanently damage the ability to learn and think creatively:

> China's stability and prosperity, and that of the region and the globe, depends on how well today's youth master the knowledge and skills that enable them to thrive in the technology-driven globalized world of the mid-21st century. Resilient public and private sector leaders of the future must be able to think creatively. Therefore, China's government should respond to population aging by acting now to invest more in the health and education of youth, especially the rural poor. (Eggleston *et al.* 2012)

India does not face China's immediate problems of an aeging population or hollowed out rural villages, but the data presented by Gaiha, Jha, and Kulkarni on the extent and severity of childhood malnutrition surely call for similar initiatives to guarantee that the next generation will have the cognitive abilities and skills to contribute to India's modernization and productivity growth.

There are many more riches in this volume than the few touched upon here. But the reader would be well advised to keep three themes in mind as the chapters are read—incomes, prices, and women's roles. These three themes provide a guide to what really matters in this volume.

Acknowledgements

This project began as a critique of an influential paper by Angus Deaton and Jean Drèze entitled: 'Food and Nutrition in India: Facts and Interpretations', published in *Economic and Political Weekly* in 2009. As our research progressed, it developed into a book. This study was funded by the British Government through its Department for Business, Innovations & Skills. We are grateful to them, especially their chief advisor, Lawrence Haddad, for their support. We are grateful to C. Peter Timmer for being a source of wisdom since the inception of this study, and for so graciously agreeing to write the *Foreword*.

Raghav Gaiha would like to thank David Bloom for the invitations to spend the summers of 2011, 2012, and 2013 at the Department of Global Health and Population (GHP), Harvard School of Public Health (HSPH). His intellectual support for this study and encouragement to explore new but related research areas have been most valuable. Support of other colleagues, Wafaie Fawzie and Peter Berman at HSPH, is also greatly appreciated. The intellectually stimulating environment at GHP not only enabled us to complete this study, but enriched it too. He would like to acknowledge his debt to K.L. Krishna, Peter Svedberg, Anil Deolalikar, and Katsushi S. Imai for their expert advice. Nidhi Kaicker deserves special thanks for being a co-author, as also for valuable contributions to other chapters.

Raghbendra Jha is grateful to his former PhD student, Anurag Sharma, at the Australian National University (ANU), for his collaboration in this research. He would like to thank ANU for providing a very conducive atmosphere for this study. He would like to thank Stephanie Hancock, in particular, for expert secretarial and administrative support, and the many colleagues at ANU who commented on many versions of the chapters in this volume both inside and outside formal seminars.

Vani S. Kulkarni would like to acknowledge with gratitude the intellectually supportive environment at the Department of Sociology, Yale University. She would like to place on record her appreciation of Professor Elijah Anderson, the William K. Lanman, Jr. Professor of Sociology at Yale University, for his academic encouragement and magnanimity in granting her time and independence to pursue scholarship; of Professor Julia Adams, Deputy Provost for Social Sciences and Faculty Development and Diversity at Yale University; and of Professor Renee C. Fox, Annenberg Professor Emerita, University of Pennsylvania, for being a source of wisdom and for enabling her to keep the value of research alive.

She expresses her deepest gratitude to her family. Her mother and (late) father, whose unconditional love and support in her academic pursuits has been a gift of life. To them, she owes all that she has today. To her dear twin sister, Veena, for her invaluable help and concern for her project and endeavours associated with it as if they were her own. To her kid sister, Varsha, whose humour and chirpiness eased the periods of stress that she experienced during the completion of this manuscript. To Angela and Swapna, who have graced her life with an extraordinary friendship, for which she remains enormously grateful.

We would like to thank the editors of *World Development*, *Applied Economics*, *Journal of Policy Modeling*, and *Journal of Asian and African Studies* for permission to reproduce published material with adaptations and extensions in this volume.

Last but not least, we owe a special debt to Raj Bhatia for his outstanding contribution as the statistical advisor.

30 June 2014

Raghav Gaiha
Raghbendra Jha
Vani S. Kulkarni

Abbreviations

AAY	Antyodaya Anna Yojana
ANU	Australian National University
APL	Above Poverty Line
ARI	Acute Respiratory Infection
ASHA	Accredited Social Health Activists
AWW	Anganwadi Workers
BD	Best District
BMI	Body Mass Index
BPL	Below Poverty Line
CDF	Cumulative Distribution Functions
CIAF	Composite Index of Anthropometric Failure
CT	Cash Transfers
CVD	Cardiovascular Disease
DALY	Disability-adjusted Life Year
FAOSTAT	Food and Agriculture Organization Statistical Databases (United Nations)
FCI	Food Corporation of India
FD	Focus District
FDI	Food Diversity Index
FGT	Foster-Greer-Thorbecke
FOD	First Order Stochastic Dominance
FPS	Fair Price Shop
GDP	Gross Domestic Product

GHP	Global Health and Population
HDPI	Human Development Profile of India
HSPH	Harvard School of Public Health
ICDS	Integrated Child Development Service
IFPRI	International Food Policy Research Institute
IHDS	India Human Development Survey
IV	Instrumental Variable
MCH	Maternal and Child Health
MDMS	Mid-Day Meal Scheme
MNC	Multinational Corporations
MPCE	Monthly Per Capita Expenditure
MSP	Minimum Support Prices
MUAC	Mid-Upper Arm Circumference
NAC	National Advisory Council
NCAER	National Council of Applied Economic Research
NCD	Non-communicable Disease
NCHS	National Centre for Health Statistics
NFHS	National Family Health Survey
NFSA	National Food Security Act
NFSB	National Food Security Bill
NGO	Non-governmental Organization
NPCDCS	National Programme for Prevention and Control of Cancer, Diabetes, Cardiovascular Diseases and Stroke
NRC	Nutrition Rehabilitation Centre
NREG	National Rural Employment Guarantee
NREGS	National Rural Employment Guarantee Scheme
NRHM	National Rural Health Mission
NSS	National Sample Survey
OLS	Ordinary Least Square
PDS	Public Distribution System
PNT	Poverty Nutrition Trap
PRI	Panchayati Raj Institution
RDA	Recommended Dietary Allowances
RHM	Rural Health Mission

RIT	Real Income Transfer
RTF	Right to Food
SAM	Severe Acute Malnutrition
SMC	School Management Committee
TPDS	Targeted Public Distribution System

1 Diets, Malnutrition, and Disease in India

An Overview

Raghav Gaiha, Raghbendra Jha, and
Vani S. Kulkarni

India is currently undergoing a rapid economic and demographic transformation. Since 1980, average living standards have experienced a sustained and rapid rise. Gross domestic product (GDP) per capita has risen by a trend rate of 4 per cent annually. Poverty declined at an annual rate of 0.88 per cent during 1983–94, and at 0.77 per cent during 1993–2004. Life expectancy rose from 54 years to 69 years while the (crude) birth rate fell from 34 per 1000 to 22 per 1000 between 1980 and 2008. Between 1980 and 2000, the share of the urban population rose from 23 to 28 per cent. By 2030, it is likely to be 41 per cent.

A key feature of the economic transformation has been the change in the nature of the Indian diet. As Indian and global markets integrate and communication improves, dietary transitions become unavoidable, resulting in a move away from inferior to superior foods, and a substitution of traditional staples by food products that are more prevalent in western diets. These shifts are reflected in higher consumption of proteins, sugars, fats, and vegetables.

Some of the underlying factors behind this dietary transition are expansion of the middle class, higher female participation in labour markets, emergence of nuclear two-income families, a sharp age divide in food preferences (with younger age-groups more susceptible to new foods advertised in the media), and rapid growth of supermarkets and fast-food outlets.

The nutritional implications of this dietary transition are, however, unclear. Recent evidence points to a 'puzzle'. Despite rising incomes, there has been a sustained decline in per capita nutrient—especially calorie intake. In an important contribution, Deaton and Dréze (2009) analyse this decline over the period 1983 to 2004. Their principal findings are:

1. Average calorie consumption was about 10 per cent lower in rural areas in 2004–5 than in 1983.[1] The proportionate decline was larger among the more affluent sections of the population, and negligible for the bottom quartile of the per capita expenditure scale. In urban areas, there was a slight change in average calorie intake over this period.
2. Proteins also experienced a drop in per capita consumption, whereas the per capita consumption of fats increased in both rural and urban areas.
3. As incomes rose over this period, these declines are puzzling. A contentious view offered by Deaton and Dréze is that the declines are not attributable to changes in relative prices. They rely on an aggregate measure of the price of food that changed little during this period. So the puzzle boils down to this: per capita calorie consumption is lower at a given level of per capita household expenditure, across the expenditure scale, at low levels of per capita expenditure as well as high; that is, there is a steady downward shift of the calorie Engel curve.[2] This implies that at the same level of expenditure in 2004, the calorie intake was lower.
4. Deaton and Dréze are emphatic that the downward shift of the calorie Engel curve is due to lower calorie 'requirements', associated mainly with better health and lower activity levels. As the evidence offered is fragmentary and patchy, but not implausible, this explanation is largely conjectural.

OBJECTIVES

The objectives of this study are to build on the Deaton and Dréze study (2009) in an attempt to resolve the nutrition puzzle by the following:

1. A detailed analysis of nutrients' intake during 1993–2004. As the broad brush treatment in Deaton and Dréze (2009) is incomplete, our analysis is designed to fill this gap, by taking into account the influences of food prices, growing affluence, urbanization, and other time-related factors such as lifestyle changes and less strenuous activity levels. The analysis allows for changes in food price elasticities over this period. This offers insights into changing consumer preferences over time.
2. As diets and nutrients' intakes are closely linked, a related objective is to throw new light on these linkages in a demand theory based analytical framework. Of particular importance is the hypothesis whether dietary diversification had a role in lowering calorie intake. While building on recent work (Economist Intelligence Unit 2012), it raises doubts about the presumption that dietary diversification is an index of diet quality, apart from throwing new light on whether it contributed to reduction in calorie intake. Related issues are pervasiveness of eating out and its nutritional implications.
3. Measurement of undernutrition using fixed nutritional norms remains contentious. A clearer understanding of the implications of different norms—whether undernutrition is alarmingly high—is crucial for policy purposes. An alternative measure that does away with these norms will also be reviewed. A point of departure of this measure is a behavioural postulate that individuals tend to switch away from the cheapest source of calories (staple food sources) after surpassing subsistence, towards more expensive sources of calories. If this switch occurs at a certain share of calories from staples, all those above the threshold are counted as undernourished (Jensen and Miller 2011).
4. Recent literature has drawn attention to poverty nutrition traps (PNTs) that limit the ability of the undernourished to engage in productive and remunerative employment. Their undernutrition persists, perpetuating their poverty. In a labour abundant agrarian economy

with a vast pool of undernourished, even a mild labour shock (for example, deficient monsoon) may impoverish large sections of the undernourished. If efficiency wage hypothesis holds, it will be harder for the undernourished to participate in employment activities and/or earn remunerative wages.

5. Another manifestation of undernutrition is child undernutrition/malnutrition, which has remained stubbornly high.[3] Most of the extant literature has focused on specific anthropometric indicators (stunting, wasting, or underweight).[4] As more than one anthropometric failure is more closely related to infectious diseases, a composite indicator and its variation will be analysed. Attention will also be given to ameliorate child malnutrition—especially through women's empowerment.
6. Among adults, growing affluence, obesity, and lifestyle changes are associated with higher prevalence of non-communicable diseases (NCDs). As there are signs of an epidemiological transition—decline in infectious disease or communicable disease mortality compensated for increasingly by higher deaths from chronic degenerative NCDs—we analyse the extent to which their growing burden is due to ageing, affluence, and overweight/obesity.[5] The policy challenge is how to address various health risks and the appropriate mix between prevention and treatment.
7. With spiralling food inflation[6] and sluggish growth of employment—especially in rural areas—the spectre of hunger and nutritional deprivation looms large for millions of households. So two major policy concerns that our study seeks to address are livelihood expansion and nutritional improvement. While National Rural Employment Guarantee Scheme (NREGS) aims to target the poor through supplementary employment in agricultural slack periods and the real income transfers have the potential for improving nutritional status, the Public Distribution System (PDS) transfers real income through a food subsidy and thus is expected to have a nutritional impact.[7] Given huge leakages from both, the magnitudes of their nutritional impact, however, need to be better assessed.
8. Much of the recent policy debate is dominated by a universal food subsidy, viewed by many as the only option consistent with a right to food, and, more contentiously, that feasible alternatives that are more universal and less targeted are likely to be more effective in

benefiting the poor. We refute these arguments on various grounds, including a perspective on the right to food that does not necessarily involve state provision of subsidized food except in emergencies, but more importantly, as a right to a right, or as a right to sensible employment and food price stabilization policies. Not just these policy choices, but also the design and scale of revamped NREGS and PDS are important questions to which simple and uncontroversial answers are unlikely.

SCHEME OF THE BOOK

Chapter 2 begins with a description of the shifts in the Engel curves for calories, protein, and fat as a prelude to a critique of the Deaton and Dréze (2009) explanation of why these shifts occurred—especially in the calorie Engel curves. Our critique is anchored to a demand theory based explanation that focuses on changes in food prices, expenditure, urbanization, and time-related factors such as sedentary lifestyles and improvements in the epidemiology of disease environment. So while the Deaton and Dréze (2009) explanation is not rejected, it is argued that it complements the demand theory based explanation. Chapter 3 focuses on dietary changes and their nutritional implications, using a two-stage instrumental variable (IV) estimation strategy.[8] First, a Food Diversity Index (FDI), analogous to the Herfindahl Index, is constructed to capture the shift away from a cereal dominated diet to more diversity in it. In the next stage, the effect of food diversity on calorie intake is analysed, controlling for the effects of various other contributory factors such as food prices, income, location, and household characteristics. If diet diversity contributes to a lowering of calorie demand, it raises doubts about the presumption that diet diversity and quality go together. As part of this dietary transition, Chapter 4 analyses pervasiveness of eating out both spatially and across different expenditure groups. Our analysis suggests that eating out is not just a middle income/expenditure class urban phenomenon, but far more pervasive. Further, as food composition and quality differ (relative to home-cooked food), there are nutritional implications. In Chapter 5, we review a recent proposal of Jensen and Miller (2011) to assess undernutrition that relies on a calorie share of staples threshold. Our analysis with the National

Sample Survey (NSS) data for 1993 and 2004 raises serious doubts about its usefulness, principally because the calorie share thresholds do not allow for the influence of any other factors except a measure of household wealth. Following important recent contributions, emphasis has shifted from low nutrition as an outcome of poverty to the former causing poverty to persist. At low levels of nutrition, workers are incapable of doing hard manual labour. Hence their productivity is low, implying low wages, low purchasing power, and therefore, low nutrition, completing a vicious cycle of deprivation. Chapter 6 identifies PNTs and assesses how pervasive they are in rural India. Under certain conditions, nutritional adequacy is a prior condition for raising incomes. Different anthropometric dimensions of child undernutrition/malnutrition (stunting, wasting, and underweight) are typically analysed separately, while children suffering from more than one anthropometric failure are more susceptible to infectious diseases (for example, diarrhoea, acute respiratory infection, etc.). A composite index of anthropometric failure is constructed, and its determinants are analysed in Chapter 7. Ageing, growing affluence and obesity, and NCDs are closely linked. In Chapter 8, we examine these using a nationwide household survey. Attention is given to complex health policy choices given the 'irreversibility' of growing affluence, lifestyle changes, and urbanization. In Chapter 9, we first analyse the real income transfers through PDS, and the reasons why these transfers are so small, followed by an examination of the (potential) contribution of NREGS and PDS in mitigating the extent and severity of undernutrition (including micronutrient deficiency).[9] From a policy perspective, and responding to the current debate on the National Food Security Bill, it is argued that a universal food subsidy is unlikely to remedy the dismal performance of the PDS, as leakages and wastages—already enormous—would be much higher. The assertion that a universal food subsidy is the only option consistent with a right to food is mistaken, as it could also be viewed as a right to a right, or as a right to sensible livelihood expansion and food policies. Chapter 10 pulls together the main findings from a broad policy perspective that draws upon lessons from policies pursued elsewhere and various initiatives in India. The vision that we construct is unavoidably 'incomplete' in some respects, but illuminates successes and failures in designing policies and in their implementation.

Our strategy here is to give the flavour of each chapter's contribution and policy implications. To avoid repetition, a consolidated policy discussion is provided in Chapter 10.

DEMAND FOR NUTRIENTS

As noted earlier, Deaton and Dréze (2009) offer an explanation of the downward shift in nutrient intake—especially calories—in terms of lower calorie 'requirements', associated mainly with better health, lower activity levels, and more sedentary lifestyles. This chapter seeks to throw more light on the decline in calorie and other nutrients' intakes and the Deaton and Dréze explanation offered from a demand theory perspective. The period (1993–2004) covered is, however, short. The analysis is carried out separately for rural and urban areas, based on data pooled over this period. The method of analysis used is robust regression.[10]

Our demand theory based explanation is valid, as food prices and expenditure have significant effects. Besides, their effects varied during 1993–2004. Over and above these effects, the time dummy[11] has a significant negative coefficient. In the context of calories, for example, it is plausible that part of the reduction in their consumption was due to health improvements and less strenuous activity levels—especially but not necessarily confined to rural areas.[12] So, while the Deaton and Dréze (2009) explanation is not rejected, it is argued that it is complementary to the demand theory based explanations.

In brief, these results confirm that the demand curve shifted over time and thus helps resolve the nutrition puzzle. As dietary transition underlies these demand shifts, it is necessary to understand the nature of this transition and the factors driving it. A better grasp of these factors would help design more effective policies to address the risks associated with diet-related non-communicable diseases (for example, cardiovascular disease, diabetes, and cancer).

DIETARY TRANSITION

This chapter analyses the dietary transition during 1993–2004, relying mostly on unit record data collected for the 50th and 61st rounds of the NSS (corresponding to 1993–4 and 2004–5, respectively).[13]

Embedding the transition in a demand theory based analytical framework, we analyse the roles of food prices, income/expenditure, socio-demographic household characteristics, location, lifestyle, and other related changes over the period 1993–2004.

While consumption of cereals, sugar, and pulses declined, there was an increase in the consumption of high-value commodities such as oil, eggs, fruits, and vegetables, and to some extent, of meat as well. As these changes are linked to intakes of calories, proteins, and fats with varying importance, an investigation of how food consumption patterns evolved in response to changes in income and relative prices is necessary.

A two-stage procedure is used to assess the impact of diet diversity on calorie demand, using the NSS data for 1993 and 2004.[14] In the first stage, we compute an FDI. This is analogous to the Herfindahl index used to measure concentration in an industry. Different food commodity shares, with 2004 prices as weights, are combined to arrive at a measure of food diversity. It ranges between 0 and 1, with higher values implying lower food diversity. Our analysis suggests that there was greater food diversity in 2004 relative to 1993. Prices, income, household size, composition, whether it belonged to the middle class, and urban location influence diet diversification.

In the second stage, using instrumental variable (IV) estimation, we analyse the effect of diet diversification on calorie demand, controlling for the effects of all explanatory variables except the middle class affiliation (consistent with IV estimation). Our results confirm that diet diversification lowers demand for calories and further contributes to a better understanding of the nutrition puzzle.

Health implications of the changes in dietary patterns are not clear-cut. There is a trade-off—while nutritionally balanced diet is associated with better health, energy dense foods are responsible for higher prevalence of NCDs such as heart disease, cancer, and diabetes.[15] Since there are some signs of an epidemiological transition in India—higher mortality from these diseases—enhancing awareness of healthy diets is important from a policy perspective.

HOW PERVASIVE IS EATING OUT?

Linked to the dietary transition is eating out. From this perspective, we give a distillation of our findings on eating out, based on an analysis of the nationwide household survey, *India Human Development Survey 2005* (IHDS), conducted jointly by the University of Maryland and the National Council of Applied Economic Research (Gaiha *et al.* 2013a). The focus is on the socio-economic status of households eating out, and their spatial distribution.[16] The latter disaggregates household locations into rural and urban areas, urban slums, and six metros.[17]

Eating out is not just a feature of metros or urban areas, but also of urban slums and rural areas. Admittedly, although it is less pervasive in urban slums and rural areas, it is non-negligible. Also, eating out is not only a feature of affluent households, as it is not uncommon among the poor and other deprived sections.[18]

Thus, eating out as a manifestation of dietary transition in India is far more pervasive than a middle-income class urban phenomenon. That this is more typical of large metros is hardly surprising, given the more rapid lifestyle changes, greater exposure to the media, and easier access to eating-out facilities. Dietary changes are also occurring in rural areas and among low-income households in response to growing affluence and the ease of eating out.

As amounts spent on eating out are conditional on a prior decision to eat out, we have experimented with the Heckman selection model.[19] In the first stage, the decision to eat out is posited to depend on household characteristics: income, type of income (salary or business), and location. In the second stage, amounts spent are attributed to most of these variables and a selection parameter (Wooldridge 2006).

Briefly, location of households, their demographic and caste characteristics, and above all, their relative affluence influence both the decision to eat out, and conditional on it, the amount spent. Affluence matters, as the effect of higher per capita expenditure (relative to the poverty line) is large and significant. Besides, the higher the share of business income, the larger is the amount spent, presumably further confirming the role of affluence in shaping preference for taste and variety in food.

Policy interventions designed to stabilize food prices and expand livelihood opportunities in rural areas thus remain an important priority 'despite' differing views on whether pervasive nutritional deprivation is real. But there are caveats to food price stabilization in a global context with some key prices (for example, vegetable oil) driven by technology and trade liberalization, and benefits of participation in NREGS greater for those with physical dexterity and stamina. The challenge of influencing food choices is a daunting one because of the complex interplay of food prices and individual preferences for taste and variety.

CALORIE THRESHOLDS AND UNDERNUTRITION IN INDIA

If we go by the per capita calorie norms of 2100 for urban areas and 2400 for the rural, the proportions of calorie deficient populations rose over the period 1993–2004, from about 58 per cent to about 64 per cent in urban areas, from about 71 per cent to about 80 per cent in rural areas, and from about 68 per cent to about 76 per cent at an all-India level. Even if lower calorie norms are used, the spectre of undernutrition looms large.

A recent contribution (Jensen and Miller 2011) is deeply sceptical of such norms for familiar reasons, and proposes an alternative measure that relies on consumption behaviour, as opposed to calorie norms.[20] This relies on the premise that individuals tend to switch away from the cheapest source of calories (staple food sources), after surpassing subsistence, towards more expensive sources of calories. All those above the calorie share of staples at which the switch occurs are counted as undernourished.

This motivated our analysis with the NSS data for 1993 and 2004, separately for rural and urban India. As the continuing food price spiral has reignited fears of another crisis with dire consequences for the poor, it is vital for policy purposes to get the measurement of undernutrition right. This concern is reinforced by a national debate on universalizing the food subsidy through the PDS.

Following Jensen and Miller (2011), we first experimented with Lowess in which the dependent variable is share of calories from cereals (cheapest and largest source of calories), and the right side variable, wealth of a household per capita, is approximated by monthly per capita expenditure (MPCE).[21]

Our estimates of undernourished are lower than those obtained using fixed calorie norms for rural and urban India. Besides, while Lowess results point to a reduction in the proportion of undernourished over the period 1993–2004—especially in rural India—a sharp rise is observed using fixed calorie cut-off points. Finally, not just lumping together of undernourished below and above the expenditure threshold, but also failure to classify those below both the expenditure and calorie share thresholds weaken the intuitive appeal of the measure of undernutrition proposed by Jensen and Miller (2011).

Following the extant literature, as also Chapters 2 and 3, establishing the important role of food prices in inducing substitutions between different sources of calories, we explore with the NSS data how sensitive calorie shares are to food prices, and whether a calorie threshold exists; and in case it does, whether estimates of undernourished change substantially. This analysis is carried out separately for the four NSS samples: rural 1993, rural 2004, urban 1993, and urban 2004, based on robust regression.

Briefly, what our analysis points to, is that the Jensen and Miller (2011) story is of limited interest and potentially misleading, principally because it confines variation in calorie share to a measure of wealth. The calorie and associated income thresholds are indeed suspect as they are influenced by several other factors—especially food prices—that are omitted. As a result, the estimates of undernourished diverge greatly.

So there is no easy way out other than to review the calorie and other nutritional norms and assess how lifestyle changes, improvements in the disease environment, reduced activity levels affect these norms, and analyse the extent and severity of undernutrition.

Are there conditions under which undernutrition affects labour market outcomes adversely, and thus perpetuates poverty? This is the subject of the next chapter.

POVERTY NUTRITION TRAP (PNT)

The effect of nutritional intake on labour productivity and wage rates, an important area of research for economists and nutritionists, found initial expression in the form of the efficiency wage hypothesis. It postulated that in developing countries, particularly at low levels of nutrition, workers are physically incapable of doing hard manual labour. Hence their productivity is low, which then implies that they get low wages, have low purchasing power, and therefore low levels of nutrition, completing a vicious cycle of deprivation. These workers are unable to save very much, so their assets—both physical and human—are minimal. This reduces their chances of escaping the PNT.[22]

The extant literature has largely ignored the impact of micronutrient deprivation on labour productivity—including the possibility of the existence of a PNT with respect to micronutrients. Our analysis is based on a nationwide household survey conducted by the National Council of Applied Economic Research in 1994.[23] We test for the existence of a PNT in the case of calories and four key micronutrients—carotene, iron, riboflavin, and thiamine—for three categories of wages (sowing, harvesting, and other), and for male and female workers separately.

The estimation procedure addresses the mutual endogeneity of both wage and nutrition. If wages affect nutrition and nutrition affects wages, they are both endogenous. An econometric test which confirms endogeneity implies the existence of PNT.[24]

We find that PNT exists in one-third (that is, ten) of the thirty cases (for example, female harvest wage and female sowing wage for calories, and both male and female workers engaged in harvesting in the case of iron). Hence, an analysis which concentrates exclusively on energy intake may present an incomplete picture of the existence of PNT.

This analysis shifts the focus to lack of nutritional adequacy as a precondition for participation in labour market activities. Even if some succeed in participating, their wage earnings will not allow them to escape the PNT. Indeed, a mild labour shock (associated with a crop shortfall) would worsen their plight, as the risk of loss of employment would be considerably higher. In particular, female workers are more prone to PNT than male workers, and there is a persistent gender inequality in rural India. We find that increasing nutrient intakes could have significant effects on rural wages and, therefore, on the possibility of breaking PNT as well as reducing poverty. Thus public policy should concentrate urgently on providing direct nutritional supplements to the nutritionally deprived in addition to pursuing direct poverty alleviation policies.

IS CHILD UNDERNUTRITION UNDERESTIMATED?

Poverty is multidimensional, and money-metric indicators such as minimum income or expenditure cannot adequately capture all these dimensions. Attention has therefore shifted to other indicators such as health status, more closely related to basic capabilities of individuals. The most commonly used anthropometric measures are stunting (low height-for-age), wasting (low weight-for-height), and underweight (low weight-for-age). Stunting is an indicator of chronic undernutrition, attributable to prolonged food deprivation, and/or disease or illness; wasting is an indicator of acute undernutrition, caused by more recent food deprivation or illness; and underweight is an indicator of both acute and chronic undernutrition. Children whose measurements fall below a certain threshold of the reference population, based on recent World Health Organization (WHO) standards, are considered undernourished: stunted, wasted, or underweight (WHO 2006a, 2006b).

An important feature of these indicators is the overlap between them, so there is a need for a more comprehensive measure of child undernutrition. Following the important work of Svedberg (2000, 2007), a new aggregate indicator is constructed that encompasses all undernourished children, be they wasted and/or stunted and/or underweight, based on IHDS. This is the composite index of anthropometric failure (CIAF).

The CIAF is about 59 per cent (or six out of ten children are undernourished). Among the subcategories, stunting and underweight, and stunting alone account for well over half of the CIAF. Children who fail in all three dimensions (simultaneously wasted, stunted, and underweight) account for a non-negligible share (13.5 per cent). Underweight alone account for the lowest share (about 6 per cent).

Recent evidence suggests that children suffering from more than one anthropometric failure are more susceptible to infectious diseases (for example, diarrhoea, acute respiratory infection) than those suffering from no failure, or just one failure. Worse, these diseases are associated with high risks of child mortality. Our analysis confirms that except for wasted and underweight and stunted only, in all other cases, the prevalence of diarrhoea was higher than in the reference group of no failure. In fact, the highest prevalence rate was among children who were simultaneously stunted and underweight, and those who were wasted, underweight, and stunted.

Our analysis of determinants of CIAF, based on robust regression, yields new insights. The larger the number of five-year-old children, the greater is the competition for food and health care, and the higher is the undernutrition. Maternal education reduces it, as it is linked to better child care and healthier diets. Quality of kitchen—whether it has a vent—contributes to more hygienic living conditions, and thus reduces CIAF. Above all, the higher the income, the lower is child undernutrition. Food prices affect child undernutrition significantly as changes in relative prices induce substitutions between food commodities and in nutrients' intakes. Of particular significance are prices of sugar, eggs, and vegetables. Lowering these prices to the extent feasible is thus likely to contribute significantly to reduction in undernutrition. Other options include strengthening of the Integrated Child Development Services (ICDS) with a mixed track record. Above all, women's empowerment is crucial to mitigate the scourge of 'nasty, brutish, and short lives' of under five-year-old children.

AFFLUENCE, OBESITY AND NON-COMMUNICABLE DISEASES

Although India lags behind other developing countries in epidemiological transition, that is, decline in infectious disease mortality compensated increasingly for by higher mortality from chronic degenerative NCDs, there is some evidence of this transition taking place.

In a comprehensive study, Mahal *et al.* (2009) demonstrate that NCDs constitute a major economic burden in India. They report high levels of out-of-pocket spending by households with members suffering from NCDs, limited levels of insurance coverage (including subsidized public services), and income losses that befall affected households. Associated with these costs are risks of catastrophic spending and impoverishment, and of course, macro impacts.

Our analysis of prevalence of NCDs is based on the IHDS 2005 conducted jointly by University of Maryland and National Council of Applied Economic Research.

We use two econometric specifications for isolating the effects of nutrient intake, socio-demographic household characteristics, and location on the occurrence of NCDs. In the first specification, our dependent variable is average prevalence of NCDs (that is, number of household members suffering from high blood pressure, or heart disease, or diabetes, or cancer/household size). In a variant, taking account of the fact that there are overlaps between various diseases (for example, between high blood pressure and heart disease, between diabetes and heart disease), and that some individuals report suffering from more than one ailment, we add up the number of ailments reported by household members and divide it by household size. As these averages cluster around zero or small values, a tobit specification is employed.[25] The unit of analysis is household.

As the demographic transition advances, and the population ages without associated improvements in living conditions, nutrition, and better access to health services, it is not surprising that ageing is a key factor in the growing burden of NCDs. Affluence also has a significant role through lifestyle changes and dietary composition. As caste affiliation better captures aspects of non-monetary deprivation, those at the bottom of the caste hierarchy (STs) have much lower prevalence of these diseases. Somewhat surprising is the low effect of overweight/obesity on NCDs. This result has to be interpreted with caution given the selective reporting of Body Mass Index (BMI) by adults.

Although the share of NCDs in the disease burden has risen, that of communicable diseases remains high, pointing to a 'double disease' burden. The shift of the disease burden toward NCDs will increase demand on the health care system. With more health care currently financed with private out-of-pocket resources, it will be increasingly harder for households to escape poverty, while more will be driven into poverty. As rural population migrates to urban areas, the associated lifestyle changes are likely to elevate NCD risks. Extreme poverty and foetal and early childhood undernutrition, from both the current situation and past exposure, are likely to create a large pool of those at elevated risk.

FOOD SUBSIDY, INCOME TRANSFER, AND THE POOR

Although rapid economic growth has led to steady progress in reducing poverty, malnutrition remains widespread, and ensuring food access for the poor remains a priority for the government. Total expenditures on food subsidies amounted to around 1 per cent of the GDP in 2009. The largest food subsidy programme is the Targeted Public Distribution System (TPDS or PDS in short), which provides households access to subsidized food staples (wheat, rice) and other items (edible oils, kerosene, sugar) (Svedberg 2012). In addition to being a food subsidy programme, the PDS serves as a minimum support price mechanism for farmers.

The objective of this chapter is to examine the reasons for low real income transfers through TPDS in three states: Andhra Pradesh, Maharashtra, and Rajasthan, based on primary data collected by the authors in 2007–8. In line with the concerns distilled from recent literature, our analysis focuses on variation in real income transfers through subsidized wheat, rice, and sugar in these states. These are associated with the poverty of a household, demographic characteristics, transaction costs of buying from PDS, food price subsidy, and (proximate) measures of supply constraints.

Given the high prevalence of undernutrition, not just in terms of calories, but also micronutrients, we also assess the nutritional outcomes of PDS relative to NREGS.

Mean real income transfer (RIT) was lowest among the acutely poor in Rajasthan; it was higher among the poor than among the moderately non-poor and (relatively) affluent; and it was highest among the (relatively) affluent in Maharashtra.

Although the determinants of RITs vary by state and food commodity, a few key determinants are emphasized below.

Land as a proximate indicator of economic status has mixed effects varying by commodity and state. Specifically, among households with owned land, RITs are higher in respect of wheat, suggesting that those better endowed benefited more in some cases. The extent of price subsidy, in most cases, results in larger RITs. Household size has a mixed effect, depending on whether economies of scale in food expenditure matter more. There is some evidence of transaction cost (distance to FPS, waiting time in a queue) limiting income gains. There is overwhelming support for supply inadequacy limiting income gains, given proximate indicators.

Our analysis highlights the extent and severity of nutritional deprivation, and the existing and potential contributions that NREGS and PDS can make towards mitigating it.

Our results, based on IV method, point to varied effects of NREGS and PDS on the intake of various nutrients. Both NREGS and PDS significantly increased the intake of calories, proteins, iron, among others, in these states. In the case of calcium, however, both PDS and

NREGS had positive and significant effects in Maharashtra, whereas neither was significant in Rajasthan. In Andhra Pradesh, on the other hand, only PDS had a significant effect on calcium consumption. These differences reflect the different ways in which income from NREGS and income transfer implicit in the PDS are spent, and the dietary preferences of households in these states.

In supplementary calculations of cost-effectiveness of NREGS and PDS, the effects vary by state and nutrient, ruling out any generalization. An implication of these findings is, however, worth emphasizing. Unconditional cash transfers touted to avoid administrative costs and corruption involved in the NREGS and PDS are likely to be much less effective if the objective is to enable large segments of the rural population to break PNT.

The case for a universal food subsidy from a right to food perspective is rejected on several grounds: direct state provision of food is not the only option consistent with this perspective except in emergencies; there is huge leakage and wastage of food under the existing TPDS which are likely to get worse; and the budgetary implications are underestimated on dubious assumptions of access and off-take.

If, instead, a revamped PDS on a much smaller scale is combined with more sensible policies that aim to augment low productivity in agriculture, avoid market imperfections that come in the way of remunerative farm gate food prices, and expand livelihood options, fulfilment of food entitlements may be far less costly. A crucial requirement is a clear enunciation of time-bound objectives and a cohesive policy framework.

POLICIES, IMPLEMENTATION, AND IMPACT

Our own evidence is viewed from a larger policy perspective that draws upon lessons from policies pursued elsewhere and various initiatives in India. The vision that we construct is incomplete, but illuminates successes and failures in designing policies and in their implementation.

Our analysis covers a large ground in resolving the nutrition puzzle, dietary diversification, child malnutrition, PNTs, prevalence of NCDs and their growing burden, and fragmented health policies.

Food prices, income, expansion of the middle class, urbanization, time-related changes in lifestyles, less strenuous activity levels, and improvement in the disease environment contributed to dietary diversification and changes in nutrient intakes. As growing affluence, urbanization, greater participation of women in the workforce are irreversible, the policy options to shape dietary diversification are limited. As markets become better integrated and supermarkets begin to drive the food policy agenda, the government's role in food price stabilization is also limited. Income augmentation through programmes such as the NREGS is constrained as the piece-rate wages tend to reward better those with greater physical stamina and dexterity. If the PNTs are pervasive, under certain conditions, nutritional adequacy is an important prior condition for the undernourished to participate in the labour market and/or earn more remunerative wages.

Child malnutrition remains stubbornly high despite rapid growth in the last two decades, pointing to the important role of factors other than income. Among these, women's empowerment has a significant role in reducing child malnutrition. Better education and employment opportunities would not only enhance their bargaining power in household decision-making, but also in ensuring that more resources are allocated to child welfare.

ICDS needs strengthening and a better coordination with National Rural Health Mission (NRHM) in tackling severe acute malnutrition (SAM).

The case for a universal food subsidy is mistaken. Nothing short of a drastic overhaul of the PDS would ensure cost-effective transfer of food to the poor.

Although the share of NCDs in the disease burden has risen and likely to rise further in the future, that of communicable diseases remains high, pointing to a 'double disease' burden. As the population ages without associated improvements in living conditions, nutrition, and better access to health services, it is not surprising that ageing is a 'key' factor in the growing burden of NCDs. Extreme poverty, and foetal and early childhood undernutrition are likely to create a large pool of those at elevated risk. The shift of the disease burden toward NCDs will increase demand on the health care system.

An important issue is whether government would play a proactive role in setting food safety standards, and in close partnership with the private sector, enforce them? Is taxation and/or subsidy an appropriate policy instrument? Could the mass media be mobilized to promote food quality when their vested interests lie elsewhere? We do not rule out effective regulation, but it would be naïve to be optimistic.

Healthy ageing is crucial for tackling NCDs.[26] Lessons learnt from developed countries point to many opportunities for their prevention and control. These relate to changes in risk levels within the population and primary care for NCDs.

What is the state of health initiatives in India? Are these based on a comprehensive system of surveillance of NCDs and expenses involved? Are public expenditure allocations in consonance with the rising burden of NCDs? Is there an overarching policy linking actions in different sectors (health, non-health)? Do different government ministries coordinate their policies towards this goal? Are there mechanisms for involving the private sector and communities in the prevention of NCDs? The concluding chapter aims to give answers to these daunting questions, even at the risk of being incomplete or sketchy.

NOTES

1. Our analysis points to some differences over the more recent period, 1993–2004, as shown in following chapters.
2. This curve denotes a relationship between calorie intake and income or expenditure. In other words, comparison of calorie Engel curves over 1993–2004 shows whether calorie intake was lower at same levels of expenditure in 2004.
3. We use undernutrition and malnutrition synonymously. The latter is defined as insufficient, excessive, or imbalanced consumption of nutrients.
4. Stunting refers to low height-for-age, wasting denotes low weight-for-height, and underweight to low weight-for-age. More precisely, stunting is measured in terms of standardized height-for-age, or z score below minus two standard deviations from median height-for-age of reference population. Algebraically, z-score = $(x_i - x_{median})/\sigma^x$. Similarly, wasting is measured as standardized weight-for-height or z score below minus two standard deviations from median weight for height of reference population. Finally, underweight is measured as standardized weight-for-age or z score below minus two standard deviations from median weight for age of reference population.
5. These diseases include cardiovascular, and diabetes, among others.
6. Spiralling inflation denotes rising inflation.
7. Real income transfers denote the transfer benefit under NREGS through wage earnings net of the opportunity cost of time spent working at constant prices.

8. Instrumental variable methods allow consistent estimation when the explanatory variables (covariates) are correlated with the error terms in a regression. See, for example, Greene (2003).
9. Under PDS, real income transfer refers to the difference between market and PDS prices multiplied by the quantity bought under PDS.
10. Robust regression is carried out when there is suspicion of heteroscedasticity in which the variance of the error term, given the explanatory variables, is not constant (Greene 2003).
11. The dummy variable takes the value 1 for 2004 and 0 for 1993.
12. With lower susceptibilty to infectious disease, absorption rate of calories is higher and their 'requirements' are lower (Deaton and Dréze 2009).
13. Our analysis broadly covers nine food commodity groups: (i) cereals; (ii) milk (including milk products, ghee, butter); (iii) oil (vanaspati oil); (iv) meat (including meat/poultry/fish); (v) eggs; (vi) pulses (including pulses, nuts, dry fruits, and others); (vii) sugar; (viii) vegetables; and (ix) fruits.
14. People buy food commodities and not calories, proteins, and fats. So the presumption here is that, if food choices are informed by their nutritional content, demand functions for nutrients are plausible (Deaton and Dréze 2009).
15. Better health denotes whether a person is physically and mentally more active and better able to participate in community life. This is linked to diet, lifestyle, and access to health care. Physical fitness is often measured in terms of body mass index (BMI), defined as an individual's body mass divided by the square of his/her height in units of kg/m^2. The normal range is (18–25) or a healthy weight-for-height. A person is classified as overweight if the BMI is in the range 25–30, and obese in the range >30.
16. As the mix of food served includes fast food (burgers, pizzas, samosas), junk food (chips, chocolate, soft drinks), instant foods (noodles, soup powder), and street foods (*chaat, tikki, golgappa*), they are high in sugar, saturated fat, salt, and calorie content, which are associated with higher risks of obesity, hypertension, and impaired glucose tolerance (Kaushik *et al.* 2011).
17. Note that these are mutually exclusive categories.
18. Both frequency of eating out and amounts spent by these deprived groups are non-negligible, as shown in Gaiha *et al.* (2013a).
19. In the Heckman model, first the probability of eating out is obtained. In the second stage, conditional on this probability, the amount spent on eating out is determined. See, for example, Greene (2003).
20. As calorie norms vary by age, sex, health status, activity patterns, and basal metabolic rate—some of which are unobservable or too difficult to measure—use of standardized norms to measure calorie deprivation is problematic. See Srinivasan (1992, 1994).

21. (a) Briefly, Lowess is used for locally weighted scatter plot smoothing. For an intuitive exposition, see Deaton (1995); (b) a logarithmic transformation of MPCE is used. For convenience of exposition, however, the logarithmic transformation is omitted.

22. For more, see Dasgupta and Ray (1986, 1987). Srinivasan (1994) offers a cogent critique.

23. For details of the survey and methodology for estimating PNT, see Jha *et al.* (2009a).

24. This is done using the Durbin-Wu-Hausman test in a regression estimated using IV method. For details, see Greene (2003).

25. In a tobit model, the dependent variable takes on 0 values with positive probability, but is roughly continuously distributed over strictly positive values (Wooldridge 2006).

26. Healthy ageing is linked to whether a person is in the normal BMI range.

2 Demand for Nutrients in India, 1993–2004*

Raghav Gaiha, Raghbendra Jha, and
Vani S. Kulkarni

Various studies point to a puzzle. In India, despite rising incomes, there has been a sustained decline in per capita calorie intake. In an important contribution, Deaton and Dréze (2009) offer a detailed analysis of the decline in calorie intake over the period 1983 to 2004. Their principal findings are summarized below.

The decline of per capita consumption is not confined to calories. It also applies to proteins and other nutrients, with the exception of fats whose consumption has increased in both rural and urban areas over this period.

As incomes rose over this period, these declines are puzzling. A more contentious view offered by Deaton and Dréze (2009) is that the latter are not attributable to changes in relative prices as an aggregate measure of the price of food—treated synonymous with the price of calories—changed little during the period in question. So the puzzle is essentially this: per capita calorie consumption is lower at a given level of per capita household expenditure, across the expenditure scale, at low levels of per capita expenditure as well as high. In other words, there is a steady downward 'shift' of the calorie Engel curve.

Deaton and Dréze (2009) are emphatic that the downward shift of the calorie Engel curve is due to lower calorie requirements, associated

* Reprinted from *Applied Economics*, vol. 45, no. 14, R. Gaiha, R. Jha, and V.S. Kulkarni, 'Demand for Nutrients in India: 1993 to 2004', pp. 1869–86, May 2013, with permission from Taylor & Francis Ltd, http://www.tandf.co.uk/journals.

mainly with better health and lower activity levels. As the evidence offered is limited, this explanation is largely conjectural.

The present study seeks to throw more light on the decline in calorie and other nutrients' intakes and the explanations offered, but over a shorter period (1993–2004). Specifically, we will first examine the changes in the pattern of food consumption and intake of calories, proteins, and fats over this period. Next, an attempt will be made to examine whether the Deaton and Dréze (2009) rejection of the role of relative prices is justified. The analysis is based on unit record data collected for the 50th and 61st rounds of the National Sample Survey (NSS) (corresponding to the years 1993–4 and 2004–5, respectively). It builds on an earlier study where the demands for calories and other nutrients were estimated using state level data. As the results for urban India were uneven, use of unit record data is likely to yield more robust results.

The scheme is as follows. We begin the chapter with comments on changes in the intake of calories, proteins, and fats during 1993–2004. An attempt is made to assess changes in the proportion of undernourished using different norms for these nutrients. This is followed by an examination of changes in Engel curves for these nutrients, and the extent to which calorie intake reduced due to lower cereal consumption. The next part discusses the specification of the demand function for various nutrients on the assumption that individuals/households are aware of nutritional value of different food commodities, and its estimation. This is followed by a discussion of the results towards the end of the chapter, focusing on shifts in demand functions over time. Concluding observations are then finally discussed.

CHANGES IN CALORIE, PROTEIN, AND FAT INTAKE

Let us first examine the changes in the distributions of calories in rural and urban areas over the period 1993–2004.

Until recently, a calorie intake of 2400 per day was considered adequate for a typical adult engaged in physically strenuous work of a certain duration in rural India.[1] More recent assessments have converged to lower calorie 'requirements' (1800).[2]

So if we use the higher calorie requirement of 2400, over 71 per cent of the rural households were undernourished in 1993 (Table 2.1).

TABLE 2.1 Calorie Intake Distributions in Rural India, 1993–2004

Year	Range of Calorie Intake Per Capita Per Day				Total
	<1800	1801–2400	2401–3000	>3000	
1993	31.09	40.07	19.42	9.42	100
	(1491)	(2084)	(2650)	(3636)	(2156)
2004	36.68	43.11	15.07	5.14	100
	(1516)	(2071)	(2629)	(3925)	(2047)

Source: 50th and 61st rounds of the NSS. Figures in parentheses are average calorie intakes.

With the lower intake of 1800, there is a sharp reduction to less than one-third of the households (about 31 per cent), implying a large concentration of households in the calorie intake range of 1800–2400. The proportion of the undernourished rises from 71 per cent to nearly 80 per cent in 2004. Also, the proportion below the lower cut-off rises from about 31 per cent to close at 37 per cent. By any standard, these imply high estimates of calorie deprivation. What is also significant is that while the mean calorie intake of those below 1800 rose slightly (from 1491 to 1516), the mean intake of the larger concentration of households in the next higher range (1801–2400) remained about the same.

Table 2.2 contains estimates for urban India. Assuming lower calorie norms of 1700 and 2100 (given less strenuous physical activity in urban areas) per day, more than a quarter of the households (about 28 per cent) consumed less than 1700 calories in 1993. More than twice this proportion (about 58 per cent) were below the higher calorie norm of 2100. Thus, well over half of the urban households were deprived in terms of calorie intake. Worse, this proportion rises to about 64 per cent over the period 1993–2004. While this is much less alarming than the calorie deprivation increase in rural India, it is nevertheless worrying.

Tables 2.3 and 2.4 contain estimates for protein intake. Following Gopalan *et al.* (1971) and Indian Council of Medical Research (1990), a cut-off of 60 (grams) of protein intake is used here. While protein deficiency is in large measure linked to calorie deficiency, it is noteworthy that well over 57 per cent of rural households consumed fewer than the required protein intake in 1993. In fact, just under a quarter

TABLE 2.2 Calorie Intake Distributions in Urban India, 1993–2004

Year	Range of Calorie Intake Per Capita Per Day				Total
	<1700	1701–2100	2101–2600	>2600	
1993	28.12	29.62	25.76	16.49	100
	(1426)	(1900)	(2320)	(3107)	(2074)
2004	29.40	34.52	24.67	11.41	100
	(1440)	(1900)	(2313)	(3252)	(2021)

Source: 50th and 61st rounds of the NSS. Figures in parentheses are average calorie intakes.

TABLE 2.3 Protein Intake Distributions in Rural India, 1993–2004

Year	Range of Protein Intake Per Capita Per Day (Grams)				Total
	<45	46–60	61–75	>75	
1993	23.81	33.79	22.79	19.61	100
	(37.1)	(52.4)	(66.8)	(94.4)	(60.3)
2004	28.81	38.05	21.46	11.68	100
	(37.4)	(52.2)	(66.3)	(93.9)	(55.8)

Source: 50th and 61st rounds of the NSS. Figures in parentheses are average protein intakes.

TABLE 2.4 Protein Intake Distributions in Urban India, 1993–2004

Year	Range of Protein Intake Per Capita Per Day (Grams)				Total
	<45	46–60	61–75	>75	
1993	24.90	37.77	23.11	14.23	100
	(37.1)	(52.4)	(66.5)	(90.7)	(57.3)
2004	29.40	34.50	24.69	11.40	100
	(37.8)	(52.3)	(66.2)	(94.9)	(55.4)

Source: 50th and 61st rounds of the NSS. Figures in parentheses are average protein intakes.

of the households consumed <45 (grams) of protein. Besides, the mean intake were well below the upper limits, implying concentration of households with relatively low protein intakes. Within both ranges of protein intake, the proportions rose more than moderately (for example, in the lower range, the proportion of households rose from about 24 per cent to about 29 per cent). However, the mean intake of protein remained unchanged. Although the share of protein-deficient urban households rose slightly (from about 62.67 per cent to about 64 per cent), the share below the lower cut-off of 45 (grams) rose more than moderately (from about 25 per cent to over 29 per cent). The mean protein intakes, however, remained unchanged in these ranges.

Tables 2.5 and 2.6 contain estimates for fat intakes. Although a precise range for fat requirements cannot be specified, Gopalan *et al.* (1971) recommends that a range of 40–60 (grams) of fat intake is desirable.[3] So even if we consider the first three ranges of fat intake, an astonishingly high estimate of fat deficiency is obtained for rural India (over 85 per cent) in 1993. In fact, well over one-third of the households are under the lowest range of <20 (grams). Over the period 1993–2004, the corresponding household share with fat intakes of <50 grams

TABLE 2.5 Fat Intake Distributions in Rural India, 1993–2004

Year	Range of Fat Intake Per Capita Per Day (Grams)				Total
	<20	21–30	31–50	>50	
1993	34.30	25.08	26.09	14.54	100
	(14.0)	(24.7)	(38.3)	(72.1)	(31.5)
2004	22.59	27.21	33.58	16.62	100
	(15.0)	(24.9)	(38.3)	(74.6)	(35.4)

Source: 50th and 61st rounds of the NSS. Figures in parentheses are average fat intakes.

TABLE 2.6 Fat Intake Distributions in Urban India, 1993–2004

Year	Range of Fat Intake Per Capita Per Day (Grams)				Total
	<25	26–40	41–60	>60	
1993	25.04	29.84	26.15	18.97	100
	(18.2)	(32.3)	(48.6)	(80.2)	(42.1)
2004	15.39	31.02	31.56	22.04	100
	(19.4)	(32.6)	(48.9)	(85.8)	(47.4)

Source: 50th and 61st rounds of the NSS. Figures in parentheses are average fat intakes.

fell but slightly (over 83 per cent). However, the share of households consuming <20 grams of fat fell sharply (from over 34 per cent to well over 22 per cent). But the mean fat intakes remained unchanged.

Using higher ranges of fat intake for urban India, fat deprivation was pervasive in urban India (about 81 per cent of the households consumed <60 grams of fats in 1993). About a quarter consumed <25 grams. Over the period 1993–2004, the reduction in the proportion of fat-deprived was barely three percentage points (from 81 per cent to 78 per cent). However, as in rural India, the proportion consuming fats <25 grams fell sharply. On the other hand, those consuming fats in the range 41–60 grams rose more than moderately. The changes in mean fat intake were negligible.

In brief, taking the norms as valid, the overall picture of nutritional deprivation worsened considerably over the period 1993–2004.

Engel Curves

CALORIES

Deaton and Dréze (2009) drew pointed attention to the downward shift in the calorie Engel curve over the period 1983–2004. Our focus is on the more recent period 1993–2004. The calorie Engel curves for rural India display a downward shift—especially above extremely low levels of monthly per capita expenditure (MPCE) at 2004 prices (Figures 2.1 and 2.2). The calorie Engel curve for 2004 crosses over the 1993 curve at (approximately) Rs 150, implying slightly higher calorie intake at lower MPCE in 2004. At higher levels of MPCE, there is a reversal with fewer calories consumed. In fact, the proportionate reduction in calorie intake is much higher at higher MPCE in 2004.

The calorie Engel curve for urban India for 2004 lies above that for 1993 up to MPCE of (a little over) Rs 500, and then below it. Thus, at MPCE <Rs 500, calorie intake was higher, and above it, lower in 2004. In fact, the proportionate reduction in calorie intake at higher MPCE was larger.

Deaton and Dréze (2009) also emphasize the reduction in calories from cereals. For rural India, the projections in Figure 2.3 illustrate the reduction in calories from cereals across all expenditure classes over the period 1993–2004. In fact, the reduction is much larger at

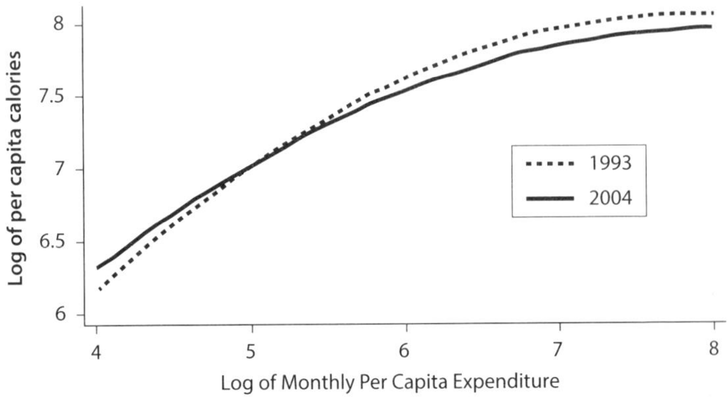

FIGURE 2.1 Calorie Engel Curves in Rural India, 1993 and 2004
Source: NSS data - Rounds 50 and 61.

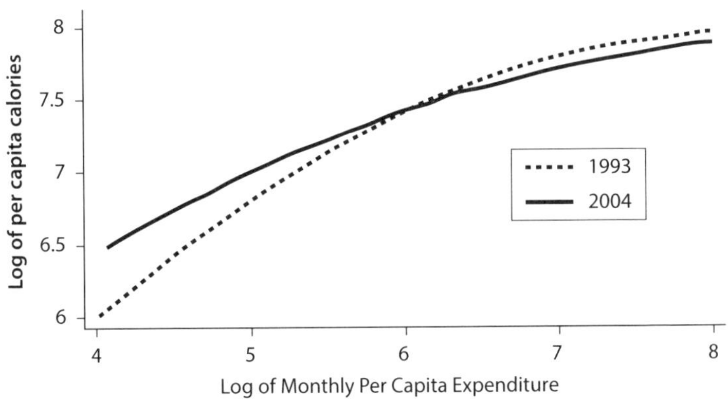

FIGURE 2.2 Calorie Engel Curves in Urban India, 1993 and 2004
Source: NSS data - Rounds 50 and 61.

higher MPCE. On average, calories from cereals reduced by 10 per cent. As cereals are the single largest source of calories, this needs investigation. In particular, we need to investigate whether cereal prices are associated with a reduction in cereal consumption, and consequently reduction in calorie intake.

Figure 2.4 for urban India presents a mixed picture, with the cereal calorie curve for 2004 lying above the 1993 curve (at about Rs 250), and below the latter at higher MPCE. So the reduction in cereal calories is a feature of higher MPCE. What is also striking is that

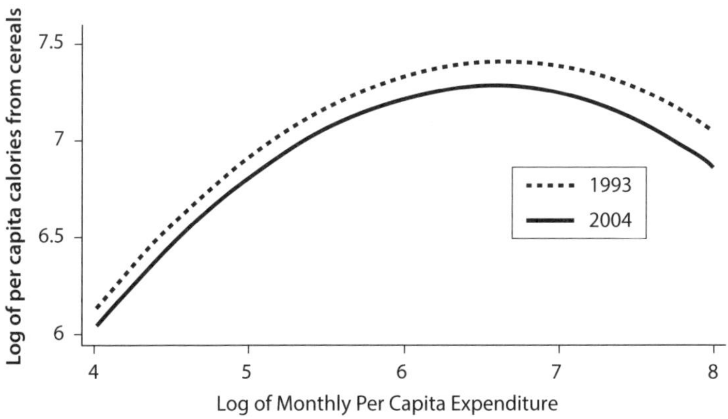

FIGURE 2.3 Calories from Cereals in Rural India, 1993 and 2004
Source: NSS data - Rounds 50 and 61.

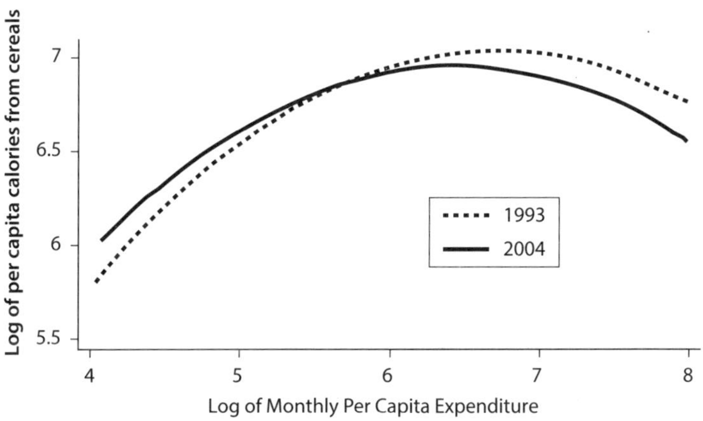

FIGURE: 2.4 Calories from Cereals in Urban India, 1993 and 2004
Source: NSS data - Rounds 50 and 61.

the reduction in cereal calories gets larger with higher MPCE. It is, therefore, not surprising that the average reduction of cereal calories is only slightly lower (over 9 per cent) relative to rural India.

PROTEIN

The protein Engel curves for rural and urban India over the period 1993–2004 are given in Figures 2.5 and 2.6. The rural–urban contrast in protein intake is striking. In the rural areas, protein intake was

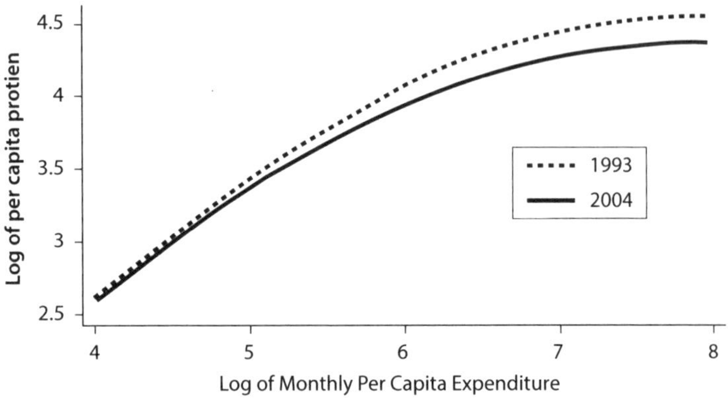

FIGURE 2.5 Protein Engel Curves in Rural India, 1993 and 2004
Source: NSS data - Rounds 50 and 61.

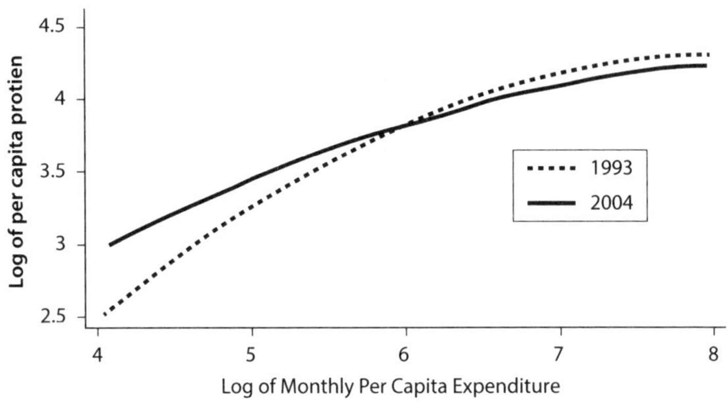

FIGURE 2.6 Protein Engel Curves in Urban India, 1993 and 2004
Source: NSS data - Rounds 50 and 61.

consistently lower across expenditure classes in 2004 than in 1993. Somewhat surprisingly, the gap between 1993 and 2004 intakes widens considerably at higher MPCE. In the urban areas, the 2004 curve was above the 1993 curve at low levels of MPCE, and after the cross-over expenditure of about Rs 500, below the 1993 curve.

FATS

The Engel curves for fats in rural India in 1993 and 2004 largely overlap, except in the higher range of expenditure, as shown in Figures 2.7

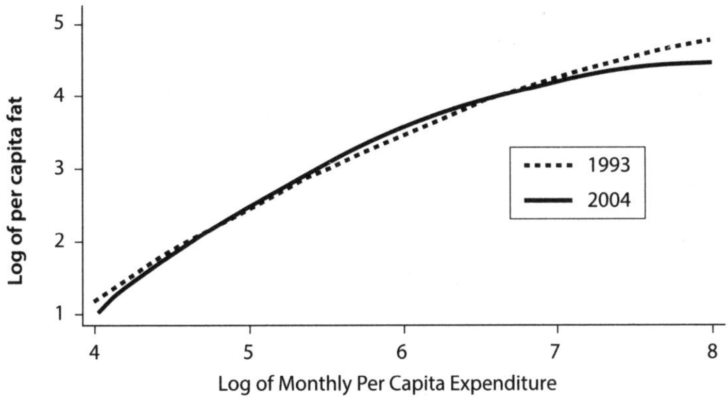

FIGURE 2.7 Fat Engel Curves in Rural India, 1993 and 2004
Source: NSS data - Rounds 50 and 61.

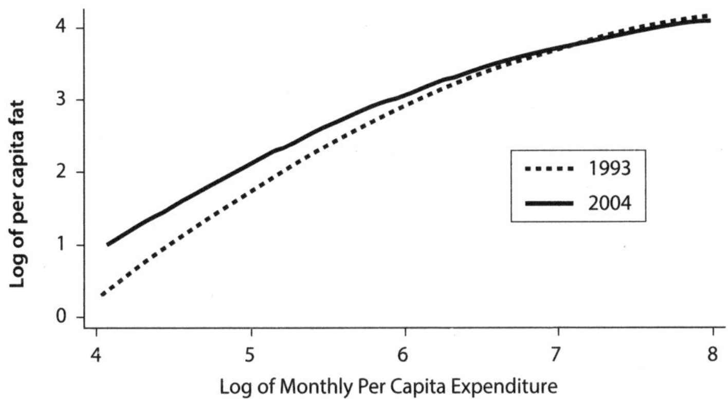

FIGURE 2.8 Fat Engel Curves in Urban India, 1993 and 2004
Source: NSS data - Rounds 50 and 61.

and 2.8. In the urban areas, by contrast, the 2004 curve lay above the 1993 curve over a large part of the expenditure scale, with a narrowing of the gap and convergence at about Rs 900.

SPECIFICATION OF DEMAND

In an earlier analysis (Gaiha *et al.* 2010b), demand equations for calories, proteins, and fats were estimated using state level data for 1993 and 2004. As the number of observations was small, and the results for urban India uneven, we aim to build on it using unit record data for rural and urban India. We expect the results to be more robust.

A basic demand equation for nutrients (calories, protein, fats) in rural and urban India with pooled data for 1993 and 2004 is given below:

$$\ln C_{it} = \alpha + \ln \mathbf{P}_{jt}\boldsymbol{\beta} + \kappa \ln E_{it} + \mathbf{X}_{it}\gamma + \lambda D_t + \varepsilon_{it} \quad (1)$$

where the dependent variable is log of nutrient consumed by ith household in time *t*; ln $\mathbf{P}_{jt}$ is a vector of log of food prices computed from the NSS at the village level (j) and time *t*; $\ln E_{it}$ is log household per capita expenditure for ith household in time *t*; $\mathbf{X}_{it}$ is a vector of household characteristics some of which are in logs (number of adult males, females, household size), others as dummy variables (caste); D_t is a dummy variable that takes the value 1 for 2004 and 0 otherwise (to allow for changes in factors other than food prices and expenditure over time); and ε_{it} is the error term. This equation is estimated using robust regression. Although a Chow test for a structural shift is not feasible with robust regression, we have employed two refinements: one is the use of a time dummy that could potentially capture the health improvements and less strenuous activity patterns (associated with easier access to drinking water, better transportation facilities), and the other is interactions of food price variables with the time dummy to allow for different price effects over time.[4]

An important point to bear in mind is that the price effects capture both own and cross-price effects through substitutions between food commodities. Briefly, as prices change, demands for commodities change, and consequently calorie (and other nutrients') intakes.

Underlying this (and other similar demand relations for protein and fats) is a presumption that food choices are informed by their nutritional content. As Deaton and Dréze (2009) emphasize, people do not buy calories and other nutrients, but food commodities. However, if food choices are informed by their nutritional values, it is meaningful to talk about demands for calories and other nutrients.[5]

RESULTS

We will first discuss the separate results for rural and urban samples for 1993, and then two sets of the pooled results for the aggregate rural and urban samples. To avoid cluttering the text with results, a selection of the results is discussed below: first separate regression results for rural and urban areas in 1993, followed by the results for rural and urban areas in 2004; and finally, the cross-sections for 1993 and 2004 with a time dummy, and then another set of pooled results with a time dummy and its interaction with food price variables.[6]

Rural India

CALORIES

Let us first consider the results on the demand for calories in rural India in 1993. The main findings are: cereal price (of rice and wheat) is negatively related to the demand for calories, while the coefficient of inferior cereals (comprising jowar, barley, bajra, millets, ragi, and other cereals) is not significant. Other food prices that reduce calorie demand are those of vanaspati oil and vegetables. Food prices that are positively associated with calorie demand are those of milk/milk products/ghee/butter, sugar, eggs, pulses/nuts/dry fruits/others. As these coefficients are elasticities, they are comparable. Cereal prices have a moderately negative elasticity, while sugar has a moderately positive elasticity. Other (absolute values of) elasticities are relatively small. Per capita expenditure (as a proxy for income) has a significant positive effect on calories demand, with a high elasticity. Household size and composition matter too. The larger the number of adult males and females, the greater is the calorie demand. Controlling for the number of adults, variation in household size reflects variation in number of children. So it is not surprising that the coefficient of household size has a significant negative effect on calorie demand. Both Scheduled Castes (SCs) and 'others' (as a residual caste group) demand more calories than the omitted group of Scheduled Tribes (STs). Education level matters too. Other things being equal, households in which adult males and females have more than middle level of schooling demand fewer calories than those with lower educational attainments.

Briefly, as expected, the estimated demand for calories is influenced by food prices and expenditure (as a proxy for income)—especially the latter—conditioned on household characteristics (including number of adults and children, educational attainments of the former, and caste affiliations).

There are, however, some striking differences between the results for 1993 and 2004. As far as food prices are concerned, a notable difference is the significant but positive coefficient of cereals. However, its elasticity is small. The coefficient of milk/milk products/ghee/butter changes, but from positive to negative. The (absolute) elasticity, however, remains low. Vanaspati oil has a significant positive coefficient in 2004, as opposed to a negative one in 1993. However, the (absolute) elasticity is much larger in 2004. Sugar retains a significant negative coefficient, but with a slightly lower value in 2004. Eggs also retain a significant positive coefficient, but with a slightly larger value. Meat/fish/poultry have a significant positive coefficient, but the value is small. Pulses/nuts/dry fruits/others retain a positive coefficient, but the value remains low. Fruits have a significant negative coefficient in 2004, but did not possess a significant one in 1993. The value of the coefficient in 2004, however, is low. Vegetables retain a significant negative coefficient, but with a slightly higher (absolute) value. Expenditure/income has a positive effect on calorie demand, but with a slightly lower value. Household size and numbers of adult males and females possess similar coefficients in 2004, as also caste affiliations. Besides, educational attainments of adult males and females have similar effects on calorie demand, as in 1993.

Briefly, while the demand function for calories is validated by significant food price and expenditure/income effects, there are significant differences in these effects between 1993 and 2004, pointing to a likely shift in the demand function.

Let us consider the results from the pooled data. While pooling has certain advantages—especially when there is panel data—a restriction is the equality of coefficients in different time periods. Our analysis of the two cross-sections for 1993 and 2004 suggests significant changes in food price and expenditure elasticities over this period, implying a (likely) shift in the demand function for calories. Accordingly, we experiment with a time dummy that acts as a shift variable and allows us to examine whether there were other changes over time (health improvements and less strenuous activity patterns) that impacted on calorie demand. This, however, is only a partial resolution of the shift in the demand function. A further refinement is therefore to check whether price elasticities changed over time by interacting the price variable with the time dummy.

The pooled results confirm significant food price effects—negative for cereals, fruits, and vegetables, and positive for inferior cereals, milk/milk products/ghee/butter, vanaspati oil, sugar, eggs, pulses/nuts/dry fruits/others. The expenditure/income effect on calorie demand is positive and large. Similar effects of household size and number of adult males and females, their educational attainments, and caste affiliations are obtained, as in the cross-section for 1993.

Over and above these effects, the time dummy has a significant negative coefficient, with a large (absolute) value, confirming that factors such as health improvements and less strenuous activity patterns may have dampened calorie demand.

The results in Table 2.7 point to significant food price interactions with the time dummy variable, confirming shifts in price effects over time. The shifts are positive for cereals, vanaspati oil, eggs, meat/fish/poultry, pulses/nuts/dry fruits/others, and negative for milk/milk products/ghee and butter, sugar, fruits and vegetables. All other effects—especially the large positive effect of expenditure—remain intact. Over and above all these, the time dummy has a significant negative effect, much larger than in the cross-section for 1993. In fact, the dummy's coefficient is larger than any of the individual price and expenditure elasticities (in absolute value). There is thus, by implication, a confirmation of the Deaton and Dréze (2009) conjecture but, without in any way diluting the demand story that we have constructed.

PROTEIN

Let us first consider the results on the demand function for protein in rural India in 1993. The main findings are: there are significant food price effects on protein demand—negative for cereals, vanaspati oil, meat/fish/poultry, fruits, and vegetables, and positive for milk/milk products/ghee/butter, sugar, eggs, and pulses/nuts/dry fruits/others. The (absolute) values of only two elasticities—cereals, and milk/milk products/ghee/butter—are high while others are small. Expenditure, however, has a significantly positive and high elasticity. Turning to household characteristics, the larger the number of adult males and females, the higher was the protein demand, while household size has

TABLE 2.7 Demand Function for Calories in Rural India, Pooled (1993–2004)

Robust Regression	Number of obs = 34371 F(29, 34341) = 390.62 Prob>F = 0.0000			
Log Per Capita Calories Intake	Coef.	Std. Err.	t	P>t
Time Dummy (0=1993, 1=2004)	−1.720	0.107	−16.010	0.000
Log prices—Rice & Wheat	−0.164	0.012	−13.450	0.000
Time Dummy × Log prices—Rice & Wheat	0.191	0.016	11.900	0.000
Log prices—Inferior Cereals	0.001	0.002	0.710	0.479
Time Dummy × Log prices—Inferior Cereals	0.004	0.005	0.820	0.414
Log prices—Milk & Milk products/ Ghee-Butter	0.027	0.004	6.110	0.000
Time Dummy × Log prices—Milk & Milk products	−0.042	0.006	−7.420	0.000
Log prices—Vanaspati oil	−0.097	0.020	−4.880	0.000
Time Dummy × Log prices—Vanaspati oil	0.285	0.026	10.800	0.000
Log prices—Sugar	0.135	0.015	9.050	0.000
Time Dummy × Log prices—Sugar	−0.037	0.021	−1.760	0.079
Log prices—Eggs	0.030	0.005	6.090	0.000
Time Dummy × Log prices—Eggs	0.054	0.010	5.570	0.000
Log prices—Meat/Fish/Poultry	−0.007	0.005	−1.380	0.168
Time Dummy × Log prices—Meat/Fish/Poultry	0.015	0.007	1.970	0.049
Log prices—Pulses/Nuts/Dry Fruits/others	0.013	0.002	5.680	0.000
Time Dummy × Log prices—Pulses	0.023	0.004	6.090	0.000
Log prices—Fruits	0.003	0.004	0.780	0.433
Time Dummy × Log prices—Fruits	−0.036	0.005	−6.870	0.000
Log prices—Vegetables	−0.085	0.007	−12.540	0.000
Time Dummy × Log prices—Vegetables	−0.041	0.010	−4.110	0.000

Log Per capita Expenditure (MPCE)	0.388	0.008	46.910	0.000
Highest Education—Male (1=above middle)	−0.024	0.004	−5.710	0.000
Highest Education—Female (1=above middle)	−0.062	0.005	−11.720	0.000
Caste—SC	0.020	0.005	4.140	0.000
Caste—Other	0.026	0.004	6.390	0.000
Log Number of adult males	0.065	0.003	18.760	0.000
Log Number of adult females	0.037	0.004	9.700	0.000
Log Household size	−0.125	0.005	−23.090	0.000
Constant	5.909	0.088	66.890	0.000
Omitted Caste: ST				

Source: Authors' calculations based on NSS (50th and 61st rounds).

a significant negative effect. In all these cases, however, the elasticities are negligibly small. The caste affiliations (SCs and 'others', relative to STs) have significant positive effects, but the coefficients are negligible. Households with adult males and females possessing above middle schooling have lower protein demands than those with lower educational attainments. Of some significance is the fact that the effect of adult males with above middle schooling is much lower than that of adult females. In sum, there is robust confirmation of a demand function with significant price and expenditure effects, conditioned on various household characteristics.

Let us now turn to the results for 2004. There are some notable differences between these and the 1993 results. While the price of cereals retains a negative coefficient, there is marked reduction in the (absolute) value of the coefficient. This is a perplexing result. While milk/milk products/ghee/butter retain a high positive coefficient, its value is smaller. Another notable difference is the change in the coefficient of vanaspati oil from a negative value to a large positive value. Sugar retains a significant positive coefficient with a slightly lower value, as also eggs, but with a larger value. The coefficient of meat/fish/poultry changes from a negative value to a positive value. The latter, however, is very small. Pulses/nuts/dry fruits/others retain a positive coefficient, but with a slightly higher value. Both fruits and vegetables have negative coefficients, with the latter taking on a larger (absolute) value. The expenditure elasticity is significantly positive, but has a lower value. Household characteristics—demographic, educational, and caste affiliations—have similar effects, as in 1993.

In brief, the changes in the price and expenditure effects point to a (likely) shift of the demand curve. So we turn to the first set of results with pooling of the cross-sections for 1993 and 2004.

With the pooling of the two cross-sections, the price effects are mostly similar (relative to, say, the 1993 results), as given in Table 2.8. There are, however, two notable differences. The coefficient of cereals is negative, but has a much lower (absolute) value. Another change is that the coefficient of meat/fish/poultry ceases to be significant. The expenditure elasticity is positive, but about the same as in 1993. The effects of household characteristics—including demographic, educational, and caste affiliations—are largely similar to those obtained with the 1993 cross-section. The effect of the time dummy is significantly negative, pointing to a shift of the protein demand curve over the period 1993–2004. The expenditure elasticity is significantly positive, but has a lower value. Household characteristics—demographic, educational, and caste affiliations—have similar effects, as in 1993.

In brief, while most of the price and expenditure effects are similar to those obtained from the 1993 cross-section, the demand function shifted.

The following interactions with time are significant: cereals (positive), milk/milk products/ghee/butter (negative), vanaspati oil (positive), sugar (negative and weakly significant), eggs (positive), meat/fish/poultry (positive), pulses/nuts/dry fruits/others (positive), fruits (negative), and vegetables (negative). Thus most price effects changed over time. The expenditure elasticity is positive and large, as in earlier analyses. Household characteristics—including demographic, educational, caste affiliations—have the same signs, but their (absolute) magnitudes are larger. Over and above these effects, the time dummy has a significant negative effect, considerably larger in (absolute) value than reported earlier. It is also larger than any of the individual price and expenditure elasticities (in absolute value).

So the conclusion is that the protein demand curve shifted as a result of price and expenditure changes—especially the former—but also because of changes in the price coefficients over time. But these

TABLE 2.8 Demand Function for Protein in Rural India, Pooled (1993–2004)

Robust regression	Number of obs = 34370 F(29, 34340) = 442.77 Prob>F = 0.0000			
Log Per Capita Protein Intake	Coef.	Std. Err.	T	P>t
Time Dummy (0=1993, 1=2004)	−2.390	0.121	−19.710	0.000
Log prices—Rice & Wheat	−0.413	0.014	−29.920	0.000
Time Dummy × Log prices—Rice & Wheat	0.381	0.018	21.020	0.000
Log prices—Inferior Cereals	−0.001	0.002	−0.550	0.581
Time Dummy × Log prices—Inferior Cereals	0.000	0.006	0.000	0.996
Log prices—Milk & Milk products	0.044	0.005	8.890	0.000
Time Dummy × Log prices—Milk & Milk products	−0.034	0.006	−5.450	0.000
Log prices—Vanaspati oil	−0.064	0.023	−2.860	0.004
Time Dummy × Log prices—Vanaspati oil	0.285	0.030	9.550	0.000
Log prices—Sugar	0.254	0.017	15.160	0.000
Time Dummy × Log prices—Sugar	−0.039	0.024	−1.610	0.107
Log prices—Eggs	0.055	0.006	9.870	0.000
Time Dummy × Log prices—Eggs	0.100	0.011	9.230	0.000
Log prices—Meat/Fish/Poultry	−0.022	0.006	−3.830	0.000
Time Dummy × Log prices—Meat/Fish/Poultry	0.036	0.008	4.290	0.000
Log prices—Pulses/Nuts/Dry Fruits/others	0.042	0.003	16.400	0.000
Time Dummy × Log prices—Pulses	0.025	0.004	5.900	0.000
Log prices—Fruits	−0.010	0.004	−2.590	0.010
Time Dummy × Log prices—Fruits	−0.033	0.006	−5.580	0.000
Log prices—Vegetables	−0.093	0.008	−12.150	0.000
Time Dummy × Log prices—Vegetables	−0.070	0.011	−6.180	0.000

(continued)

TABLE 2.8 Continued

Robust regression	Number of obs = 34370 F(29, 34340) = 442.77 Prob>F = 0.0000			
Log Per Capita Protein Intake	Coef.	Std. Err.	T	P>t
Log Per capita Expenditure (MPCE)	0.452	0.009	48.460	0.000
Highest Education—Male (1=above middle)	−0.026	0.005	−5.570	0.000
Highest Education—Female (1=above middle)	−0.066	0.006	−11.020	0.000
Caste—SC	0.033	0.006	6.030	0.000
Caste—Other	0.029	0.005	6.120	0.000
Log Number of adult males	0.056	0.004	14.150	0.000
Log Number of adult females	0.024	0.004	5.620	0.000
Log Household size	−0.077	0.006	−12.600	0.000
Constant	1.827	0.100	18.340	0.000
Omitted Caste: ST				

Source: Authors' calculations based on NSS (50th and 61st rounds).

effects were set against the effects of other factors that impinged on protein demand, but were unrelated to price and expenditure changes.

FATS

Let us first consider the results obtained for rural India 1993.

The main findings are: the price of cereals has a negative effect on fat demand, and the (absolute) value is large. So do inferior cereals, but the (absolute) value is low. Milk/milk products/ghee/butter have a significant negative coefficient, but the (absolute) value is small. Vanaspati oil has a significant positive effect with a moderate value of the coefficient. Sugar has a significant positive effect and the elasticity is high. Eggs too have a significant positive effect, but the value is small. Meat/fish/poultry have a positive effect, but the coefficient is small. Pulses/nuts/dry fruits/others have a significant positive coefficient, and its value is moderate. Fruits have a positive coefficient, but the value is small, as also vegetables, but the coefficient of the latter is larger. The elasticity of expenditure is much larger than that for calories. Household size has no significant effect, but numbers of adult males and females have significant positive effects. The coefficients, however, are negligibly small. Castes (SC and 'others', relative to ST) have significant positive effects, but the coefficients are negligible. While households with adult males possessing above middle school education have higher fat demand, there is a reversal of this effect with adult females. The coefficient of the latter, however, is negligible. In brief, the existence of a demand function with strong food price and expenditure effects is corroborated, conditioned on various household characteristics.

There are some notable differences between the 1993 and 2004 food price effects. Cereals have a significant positive coefficient in 2004, while in 1993 it was negative with a large (absolute) value. There is also a sign reversal for inferior cereals, with a positive coefficient in 2004, but the value of the coefficient is small. The sign of milk/milk products/ghee/butter remains negative, but the (absolute) value is much larger, as also of vanaspati oil. Sugar retains a positive coefficient, but with a considerably smaller value. Eggs, by contrast, retain a positive coefficient, but with a larger value. Meat/fish/poultry retain a positive coefficient, but with a larger value, as also pulses/nuts/dry fruits/others. Fruits, by contrast, retain a positive but smaller coefficient, as also vegetables. The expenditure elasticity is positive, but smaller than in 1993. All household characteristics (including household size which did not possess a significant coefficient in 1993), except adult males with over middle level schooling (significant in 1993) and number of adult females (significant in 1993). In most cases, however, the coefficients are negligible except 'others' as the residual caste group. In brief, the evidence points to a (likely) shift in the demand curve for fats in rural India.

Let us now compare the pooled results for rural India in Table 2.9 with those for 1993. Beginning with the food price effects, cereal price has a negative coefficient but the value is considerably smaller. Inferior cereals cease to have a significant coefficient. Milk/milk products/ghee/butter retain a negative coefficient, but with a larger (absolute value). Vanaspati oil, by contrast, retains a negative coefficient but with a larger (absolute) value. Sugar retains a positive coefficient, but with a smaller value. Eggs also retain a positive coefficient, but with a slightly larger value. Meat/fish/poultry retain a positive but slightly larger coefficient, as also pulses/nuts/dry fruits/others. Fruits have a positive coefficient, but with little change in its value, as also vegetables. The elasticity of expenditure remains significantly positive but the value is lower. While all household characteristics other than the number of adult females have significant coefficients, the values are negligible. Over and above these effects, the dummy has a significant negative coefficient, suggesting a downward shift of the fat demand curve due to factors other than those specified in the demand function over time. The important point is that the value of the coefficient is large.

All food prices and time dummy interactions are significant, implying changes in price elasticities over the period 1993–2004. Negative interactions are found for milk/milk products/ghee/butter, vanaspati oil, sugar, and vegetables. On the other hand, positive interactions are observed for cereals, inferior cereals, eggs, meat/fish/poultry, and pulses/nuts/dry fruits/others. The expenditure elasticity is positive and high. The effect of number of adult males is positive, while that of household size is negative.

Number of adults with over middle level schooling has a positive effect while that of females is negative. All these effects are, however, small. Castes, on the other hand, have significant positive effects (relative to STs). The effect of the time dummy is positive and large.

Thus there is additional support for a shift in the demand function for fats in rural India.

Urban India

CALORIES

Let us first consider the results for urban India in 1993. With the exceptions of vanaspati oil and meat/fish/poultry, all other prices had significant demand effects. These include a negative effect of cereals, but small in (absolute) value; inferior cereals had a weakly significant effect but the (absolute) value was negligible; milk/milk products/ghee/butter had a positive effect but the coefficient was small; sugar had a moderately positive effect; eggs had a positive but small effect; pulses/nuts/dry fruits/others had a small positive effect; and both fruits and vegetables had negative effects but small in (absolute)

TABLE 2.9 Demand Function for Fats in Rural India, Pooled (1993–2004)

Robust regression	Number of obs = 34371 F(29, 34341) = 772.70 Prob>F = 0.0000			
Log Per Capita Fat Intake	Coef.	Std. Err.	t	P>t
Time Dummy (0=1993, 1=2004)	0.651	0.196	3.320	0.001
Log prices—Rice & Wheat	−0.565	0.022	−25.380	0.000
Time Dummy × Log prices—Rice & Wheat	0.610	0.029	20.840	0.000
Log prices—Inferior Cereals	−0.012	0.004	−3.370	0.001
Time Dummy × Log prices—Inferior Cereals	0.066	0.009	7.280	0.000
Log prices—Milk & Milk products	−0.042	0.008	−5.270	0.000
Time Dummy × Log prices—Milk & Milk products	−0.151	0.010	−14.800	0.000
Log prices—Vanaspati oil	0.088	0.036	2.410	0.016
Time Dummy × Log prices—Vanaspati oil	−0.455	0.048	−9.450	0.000
Log prices—Sugar	0.531	0.027	19.600	0.000
Time Dummy × Log prices—Sugar	−0.388	0.039	−10.050	0.000
Log prices—Eggs	0.068	0.009	7.460	0.000
Time Dummy × Log prices—Eggs	0.095	0.018	5.430	0.000
Log prices—Meat/Fish/Poultry	0.051	0.009	5.610	0.000
Time Dummy × Log prices—Meat	0.063	0.013	4.670	0.000
Log prices—Pulses/Nuts/Dry Fruits/others	0.110	0.004	26.410	0.000
Time Dummy × Log prices—Pulses	0.062	0.007	9.080	0.000
Log prices—Fruits	0.026	0.006	3.990	0.000
Time Dummy × Log prices—Fruits	−0.009	0.010	−0.960	0.338
Log prices—Vegetables	0.183	0.012	14.760	0.000
Time Dummy × Log prices—Vegetables	−0.132	0.018	−7.220	0.000

(continued)

TABLE 2.9 Continued

Robust regression	Number of obs = 34371 F(29, 34341) = 772.70 Prob>F = 0.0000			
Log Per Capita Fat Intake	Coef.	Std. Err.	t	P>t
Log Per capita Expenditure (MPCE)	0.858	0.015	56.930	0.000
Highest Education—Male (1=above middle)	0.021	0.008	2.800	0.005
Highest Education—Female (1=above middle)	−0.050	0.010	−5.130	0.000
Caste—SC	0.132	0.009	14.720	0.000
Caste—Other	0.206	0.008	27.330	0.000
Log Number of adult males	0.023	0.006	3.560	0.000
Log Number of adult females	0.009	0.007	1.310	0.190
Log Household size	−0.033	0.010	−3.330	0.001
Constant	−2.949	0.161	−18.310	0.000
Omitted Caste: ST				

Source: Authors' calculations based on NSS (50th and 61st rounds).

values—especially that of fruits. The expenditure elasticity was positive and high. Out of the household characteristics, except for the caste variables, all others were significant, but small in values. In brief, the evidence in support of a demand function for calories in urban India in 1993 is robust, with significant price and expenditure effects.

In 2004, the expenditure elasticity is positive but lower. Household size has a negative coefficient while number of adult males and females have positive coefficients. However, these effects are negligible. Both educational variables have significant negative coefficients, with that of adult males small in (absolute) value and that of adult females negligible. There are some striking changes in the price effects. Cereals retain a negative coefficient with little change in its value; inferior cereals cease to be significant, as also milk/milk products/ghee/butter; vanaspati oil has a significant positive coefficient with a moderately high elasticity (not significant in 1993); sugar retains a positive (weakly significant) coefficient, but lower in value; eggs retain a positive coefficient with a much larger value; meat/fish/poultry had a significant positive coefficient, but small in value (not significant in 1993); pulses/nuts/dry fruits retain a positive but small coefficient; fruits retain a negative coefficient with a small (absolute) value; and vegetables, by contrast, retain a negative coefficient, but larger in (absolute) value. There is, thus, a robust confirmation of the demand function for calories in urban India in 2004. As before, our comments are confined to a comparison of the pooled results with those for 1993.

One notable difference is that all price effects are significant in 2004. Both cereals and inferior cereals have negative coefficients, but small in (absolute) value. Milk/milk products/ghee/butter retain a positive coefficient, but with a low value. Vanaspati oil has a positive effect with a moderately higher coefficient. Sugar retains a positive coefficient with a similar value. Eggs also retain a positive coefficient with a slightly larger value. Meat/fish/poultry have a weakly significant coefficient with a small value. Pulses/nuts/dry fruits/others retain a small positive coefficient. Fruits have a negative coefficient, but small in (absolute) value, as also vegetables. The expenditure elasticity is positive, but much lower. Excluding the caste variables, all other household characteristics have significant coefficients, but they are negligible in value. Over and above these effects, the time dummy has a significant negative coefficient. As the (absolute) value is large, it follows that there were shift factors not unlike those conjectured for rural India. In brief, the demand function shifted over time.

Turning to the results with food price and time interactions in Table 2.10, there is ample evidence of a shift in the demand curve for calories.

Except for inferior cereals, meat/fish/poultry, and fruits, all other food prices had significant interaction effects, implying changes in price elasticities over time. These include cereals (negative), milk (negative), vanaspati oil (positive), sugar (negative), eggs (positive), fruits (negative), and vegetables (negative). The time dummy has a significant negative effect with a large (absolute) value. In fact, it is much larger (in absolute value) than any individual price and expenditure elasticities. The expenditure elasticity is moderately high. Except for the caste variables and education of adult males, all other household characteristics have significant but small coefficients. In brief, the demand curve shifted over time.

TABLE 2.10 Demand Function for Calories in Urban India, Pooled (1993–2004)

Robust regression	Number of obs = 24803 F(29, 24773) = 409.12 Prob>F = 0.0000			
Log Per Capita Calories Intake	Coef.	Std. Err.	t	P>t
Time Dummy (0=1993, 1=2004)	−0.920	0.119	−7.730	0.000
Log prices—Rice & Wheat	−0.051	0.013	−3.820	0.000
Time Dummy × Log prices—Rice & Wheat	−0.036	0.018	−2.000	0.045
Log prices—Inferior Cereals	−0.003	0.002	−1.490	0.135
Time Dummy × Log prices—Inferior Cereals	−0.004	0.005	−0.790	0.429
Log prices—Milk & Milk products/Ghee/Butter	0.023	0.006	3.910	0.000
Time Dummy × Log prices—Milk & Milk products	−0.023	0.009	−2.550	0.011
Log prices—Vanaspati oil	−0.010	0.023	−0.420	0.675
Time Dummy × Log prices—Vanaspati oil	0.226	0.030	7.500	0.000
Log prices—Sugar	0.107	0.018	5.930	0.000
Time Dummy × Log prices—Sugar	−0.084	0.026	−3.240	0.001
Log prices—Eggs	0.034	0.007	4.630	0.000
Time Dummy × Log prices—Eggs	0.105	0.015	6.960	0.000
Log prices—Meat/Fish/Poultry	0.000	0.006	0.020	0.984
Time Dummy × Log prices—Meat/Fish/Poultry	0.007	0.008	0.880	0.380
Log prices—Pulses/Nuts/Dry Fruits/others	0.014	0.003	4.400	0.000
Time Dummy × Log prices—Pulses	0.004	0.005	0.700	0.487
Log prices—Fruits	−0.007	0.005	−1.540	0.124
Time Dummy × Log prices—Fruits	−0.031	0.008	−3.990	0.000
Log prices—Vegetables	−0.038	0.008	−4.950	0.000
Time Dummy × Log prices—Vegetables	−0.079	0.012	−6.430	0.000

Log Per capita Expenditure (MPCE)	0.282	0.012	23.980	0.000
Highest Education—Male (1=above middle)	−0.008	0.006	−1.360	0.175
Highest Education—Female (1=above middle)	−0.027	0.006	−4.720	0.000
Caste—SC	−0.006	0.008	−0.680	0.498
Caste—Other	−0.008	0.007	−1.150	0.250
Log Number of adult males	0.084	0.004	21.520	0.000
Log Number of adult females	0.042	0.004	10.030	0.000
Log Household size	−0.193	0.009	−21.850	0.000
Constant	5.978	0.118	50.840	0.000
Omitted Caste: ST				

Source: Authors' calculations based on NSS (50th and 61st rounds).

PROTEIN

Let us first comment on the demand equation for protein in urban India for 1993. All price effects are significant. Cereals have a negative effect, as also inferior cereals, with the coefficient of the former much larger in (absolute) value. Milk/milk products/ghee/butter have a small positive effect. Sugar has a moderately high positive effect, as also eggs, but with a small coefficient. Meat/fish/poultry have a negative effect, but with a small (absolute) value. Pulses/nuts/dry fruits/others have a positive bur small effect. Fruits have a negative effect with a small (absolute) value, as also vegetables. The expenditure elasticity is high. Except for the caste variables, all other household characteristics have significant effects. Household size and number of adult males and females have significant effects, but the values are negligible. While educational levels of adult males and females have significant effects, that of the former is small while that of the latter is negligible. Thus the demand function for protein in urban India in 1993 is robust, given the significant price and expenditure effects.

Let us now compare the results for 2004 with those for 1993. All food price effects for 2004 are significant. Cereals have a negative coefficient but smaller in (absolute) value; inferior cereals also have a negative coefficient but the (absolute) value is very small; milk/milk products/ghee/butter retain a positive coefficient, but with a slightly lower value; vanaspati oil has a significant positive coefficient with a high value (not significant in 1993); sugar has a positive coefficient but smaller in value; eggs retain a positive coefficient, but the value is larger; meat/fish/poultry have a negative coefficient, but with a small (absolute) value; pulses/nuts/dry fruits/others retain a positive coefficient with a similar value; and both fruits and vegetables retain negative coefficients with the (absolute) value of the latter larger. The expenditure elasticity is positive, but much lower. Out of the household variables, all (except 'others' as the second caste variable) have significant coefficients, but in most cases, these are either very small or negligible. In brief, the evidence suggests significant changes in food price and expenditure effects.

In order to confirm that there was a shift in the demand curve, we experiment with a time dummy. The results are given in Table 2.11. These are compared with the results for 1993.

Cereal price retains a negative coefficient, but the (absolute) value is lower; inferior cereals retain a negative coefficient but with a slightly larger (absolute) value. Milk/milk products/ghee/butter retain a positive coefficient with a similar value. Vanaspati oil has a significant coefficient with a moderately high value (not significant in 1993). Sugar retains a positive coefficient, but the value is slightly lower. Eggs retain a positive coefficient, but with a slightly larger value. Meat/fish/poultry retain a negative coefficient with a small (absolute) value. Pulses retain a small positive coefficient. Fruits retain a negative coefficient with a small (absolute) value. Vegetables, by contrast, retain a negative coefficient, but with a slightly larger (absolute) value. The expenditure elasticity is high but lower. Except for SCs (with a small positive coefficient), all other household variables have significant coefficients, but negligible in value. The time dummy has a negative coefficient, and it is large in (absolute) value, implying a shift in the demand curve.

Except for pulses/nuts/dry fruits/others, all other food prices' interactions with time were significant, implying changes in food price elasticities over time. Briefly, the interactions were significant for cereals (positive), inferior cereals (negative), milk/milk products/ghee/butter (negative), vanaspati oil (positive), sugar (negative), eggs (positive), meat/fish/poultry (positive), fruits (negative), and vegetables (negative). The time dummy has a negative coefficient. Also, it is larger

TABLE 2.11 Demand Function for Protein in Urban India, Pooled (1993–2004)

Robust regression	Number of obs = 24803 F(`, 24773) = 384.72 Prob>F = 0.0000			
Log Per Capita Protein Intake	Coef.	Std. Err.	t	P>t
Time Dummy (0=1993, 1=2004)	−1.340	0.131	−10.250	0.000
Log prices—Rice & Wheat	−0.232	0.015	−15.940	0.000
Time Dummy × Log prices—Rice & Wheat	0.095	0.020	4.740	0.000
Log prices—Inferior Cereals	−0.005	0.002	−2.370	0.018
Time Dummy × Log prices—Inferior Cereals	−0.016	0.005	−2.990	0.003
Log prices—Milk & Milk products/Ghee/Butter	0.050	0.006	7.730	0.000
Time Dummy × Log prices—Milk & Milk products	−0.026	0.010	−2.560	0.010
Log prices—Vanaspati oil	0.032	0.025	1.270	0.206
Time Dummy × Log prices—Vanaspati oil	0.252	0.033	7.620	0.000
Log prices—Sugar	0.258	0.020	12.930	0.000
Time Dummy × Log prices—Sugar	−0.102	0.028	−3.580	0.000
Log prices—Eggs	0.057	0.008	7.130	0.000
Time Dummy × Log prices—Eggs	0.142	0.017	8.590	0.000
Log prices—Meat/Fish/Poultry	−0.041	0.006	−6.670	0.000
Time Dummy × Log prices—Meat/Fish/Poultry	0.016	0.009	1.770	0.077
Log prices—Pulses/Nuts/Dry Fruits/others	0.039	0.004	11.010	0.000
Time Dummy × Log prices—Pulses	0.003	0.006	0.610	0.543
Log prices—Fruits	−0.018	0.005	−3.290	0.001
Time Dummy × Log prices—Fruits	−0.041	0.009	−4.840	0.000
Log prices—Vegetables	−0.019	0.008	−2.220	0.027

(continued)

TABLE 2.11 Continued

Robust regression	Number of obs = 24803 F(29, 24773) = 384.72 Prob>F = 0.0000			
Log Per capita Protein Intake	Coef.	Std. Err.	t	P>t
Time Dummy × Log prices—Vegetables	−0.127	0.013	−9.450	0.000
Log Per capita Expenditure (MPCE)	0.327	0.013	25.290	0.000
Highest Education—Male (1=above middle)	−0.018	0.006	−2.920	0.003
Highest Education—Female (1=above middle)	−0.033	0.006	−5.260	0.000
Caste—SC	0.023	0.009	2.500	0.013
Caste—Other	0.009	0.008	1.090	0.276
Log Number of adult males	0.077	0.004	18.070	0.000
Log Number of adult females	0.031	0.005	6.760	0.000
Log Household size	−0.147	0.010	−15.110	0.000
Constant	1.823	0.129	14.120	0.000
Omitted Caste: ST				

Source: Authors' calculations based on NSS (50th and 61st rounds).

(in absolute) value than individual price or expenditure elasticities. There is no change in the expenditure elasticity.

In sum, the shift in the demand curve for protein reflected changes in food price elasticities and other factors that changed over time.

FATS

The analysis of demand for fats using state level data in Gaiha *et al.* (2010b) did not yield satisfactory results. With household data, the results are stronger. Let us first comment on the food price effects on the demand for fats in urban India in 1993.

Cereal price has a negative effect on fat demand, and the value of the coefficient is large. Milk/milk products/ghee/butter have a negative effect with a small (absolute) value of the coefficient. Vanaspati oil has a positive effect with a moderately large coefficient. Sugar, too, has a positive effect with a large value of the coefficient. Eggs, by contrast, have a positive effect, but the coefficient is small. Meat/fish/poultry have a positive effect, but the size is small. Pulses/nuts/dry fruits/others also have a positive effect, but the size is moderate. Vegetables have a positive effect and the size is large. The expenditure elasticity is high. While all household variables—except household size—have significant effects, the effect associated with 'others' as a residual caste group is positive and large. In brief, strong food price and expenditure effects corroborate a robust demand function for fats in urban India in 1993.

There are some striking differences between the 1993 and 2004 results. Cereal price ceases to have a significant effect while that of inferior cereals has a negative effect (not significant in 1993) with a small (absolute) value. Milk/milk products/ghee/butter retain a negative coefficient with a larger (absolute) value. Vanaspati oil changes sign from positive to negative and the coefficient has a moderate (absolute) value. Sugar retains a positive coefficient, but with a smaller value. Eggs, however, retain a positive coefficient, but with a considerably larger value. Meat/fish/poultry also retain a positive coefficient, but with a slightly larger value. Pulses/nuts/dry fruits/others retain a positive coefficient, but with a considerably lower value. The expenditure elasticity drops sharply. All household variables have significant coefficients, but only two are small (education of adult males) or large ('others' as a residual caste group). While a demand function is corroborated by significant food price and expenditure effects, the changes over time are of some importance, as our subsequent analysis suggests.

Let us now compare the pooled sample results in Table 2.12 with those for 1993. There are, again, some striking differences. Cereal price retains a negative coefficient, but with a smaller (absolute) value. Inferior cereals have a weakly significant negative coefficient (not significant in 1993) and the (absolute) value is negligible. Milk/milk products/ghee/butter retain a negative coefficient, but with a slightly larger (absolute) value. Vanaspati oil retains a positive coefficient, but with a considerably lower value. Sugar retains a positive coefficient, but with a slightly lower value. Eggs also retain a positive coefficient, but with a larger value. Meat/fish/poultry retain a positive coefficient with a slightly larger value; pulses/nuts/dry fruits/others retain an unchanged positive coefficient; vegetables retain a positive coefficient with a slightly lower value. The expenditure elasticity is high, but considerably lower than

TABLE 2.12 Demand Function for Fats in Urban India, Pooled (1993–2004)

Robust regression	Number of obs = 24802 F(29, 24772) = 740.76 Prob> F = 0.0000			
Log Per Capita Fat Intake	Coef.	Std. Err.	T	P>t
Time Dummy (0=1993, 1=2004)	0.663	0.202	3.280	0.001
Log prices—Rice & Wheat	−0.271	0.023	−12.020	0.000
Time Dummy × Log prices—Rice & Wheat	0.253	0.031	8.180	0.000
Log prices—Inferior Cereals	0.002	0.003	0.500	0.615
Time Dummy × Log prices—Inferior Cereals	−0.030	0.008	−3.740	0.000
Log prices—Milk & Milk products/Ghee/Butter	−0.025	0.010	−2.460	0.014
Time Dummy × Log prices—Milk & Milk products	−0.103	0.016	−6.570	0.000
Log prices—Vanaspati oil	0.229	0.039	5.880	0.000
Time Dummy × Log prices—Vanaspati oil	−0.376	0.051	−7.350	0.000
Log prices—Sugar	0.503	0.031	16.340	0.000
Time Dummy × Log prices—Sugar	−0.291	0.044	−6.620	0.000
Log prices—Eggs	0.030	0.012	2.410	0.016
Time Dummy × Log prices—Eggs	0.223	0.026	8.690	0.000
Log prices—Meat/Fish/Poultry	0.036	0.010	3.740	0.000
Time Dummy × Log prices—Meat/Fish/Poultry	0.023	0.014	1.600	0.110
Log prices—Pulses/Nuts/DryFruits/others	0.164	0.006	29.840	0.000
Time Dummy × Log prices—Pulses	−0.046	0.009	−5.390	0.000
Log prices—Fruits	0.003	0.008	0.380	0.702
Time Dummy × Log prices—Fruits	−0.002	0.013	−0.140	0.887
Log prices—Vegetables	0.300	0.013	23.070	0.000
Time Dummy × Log prices—Vegetables	−0.128	0.021	−6.120	0.000

Log Per capita Expenditure (MPCE)	0.748	0.020	37.450	0.000
Highest Education—Male (1=above middle)	−0.007	0.009	−0.740	0.462
Highest Education—Female (1=above middle)	−0.047	0.010	−4.760	0.000
Caste—SC	0.293	0.014	20.570	0.000
Caste—Other	0.311	0.012	25.550	0.000
Log Number of adult males	0.037	0.007	5.560	0.000
Log Number of adult females	0.032	0.007	4.510	0.000
Log Household size	−0.054	0.015	−3.570	0.000
Constant	−3.536	0.200	−17.700	0.000
Omitted Caste: ST				

Source: Authors' calculations based on NSS (50th and 61st rounds).

in 1993. All household variables, with the exception of SCs, have significant effects, but negligible in value. SCs demand more fats relative to STs. That the demand function shifted is reflected in the negative coefficient of the time dummy. The (absolute) value of the coefficient is large.

All price and time interaction effects, except for fruits, are significant, implying that price elasticities changed over the period 1993–2004. Specifically, the interaction effects are: cereals (positive), inferior cereals (negative), milk/milk products/ghee/butter (negative), vanaspati oil (negative), sugar (negative), eggs (positive), meat/fish/poultry (positive but weakly significant), pulses/nuts/dry fruits/others (negative), and vegetables (negative). The time dummy coefficient sign changes from negative to positive, implying a shift due to factors not specified in the demand function (for example, eating out). Also, it is large. The expenditure elasticity is positive (and about the same as with the pooled sample without interactions).

So the demand function shifted over time.

***

In an influential study, Deaton and Dréze (2009) drew attention to a puzzle: despite rising incomes, there has been a sustained decline in per capita calorie intake over the period 1983–2004—especially in rural areas. Specifically, per capita consumption of calories is lower at a given level of per capita household expenditure, across the expenditure scale, at low levels of per capita expenditure as well as high. In other words, there is a steady downward shift of the calorie Engel curve. Further, the decline is not confined to calories. It applies to protein and other nutrients, with the exception of fats, whose consumption has increased in both rural and urban areas. They are emphatic that the downward shift of the calorie Engel curve is due to lower calorie requirements, associated mainly with better health and lower and less strenuous activity levels.

We have developed an alternative explanation of changes in the consumption of calories, protein, and fats over the more recent period, 1993–2004. This explanation is embedded in a standard demand theory framework, with food prices and expenditure (as a proxy for income) cast in a pivotal role. Based on different experiments, robust demand functions are estimated for each of three nutrients, viz. calories, protein, and fats, separately for rural and urban areas. Our results show consistently robust food price and expenditure effects. Besides, shifts in food price elasticities over time are significant. Over and above these effects, there are shifts in demands due to factors other than those specified in the demand equations. In the context of calories, for example, it is plausible that part of the reduction in their consumption was due to health improvements and less strenuous activity levels—especially, but not necessarily confined to, rural areas.

In conclusion, while the Deaton and Drèze (2009) explanation is not rejected; it is arguable that it is complementary to the demand-based explanations.

NOTES

1. In conformity with convention, we use average calorie norm. Even this has been questioned on various grounds, but the consensus view is that they are much lower than the norm of 2400 per day. See, for example, FAO's SOFI 2012.
2. Srinivasan (1992) is deeply skeptical of such requirements on the grounds that energy expenditure adjusts to intake within a range.
3. Gopalan *et al.* (1971) observe 'The quantity of fat that should be included in a well-balanced diet is not known with any degree of certainty. However, it

appears desirable in the present state of knowledge that the daily intake of fat should be such that it contributes no more than 15 to 20 per cent of the calories in the diet. A total of about 40 to 60 gms of fat can therefore be safely consumed daily, and in order to obtain the necessary amounts of essential fatty acids, the fat intake should include at least 15 gms of vegetable oils' (p. 8).

4. This specification is not restrictive as it allows both the intercept and slopes to vary with time.

5. See, for example, Pitt (1983), Pitt and Rosenzweig (1985), and Behrman and Deolalikar (1988).

6. Separate cross-section results for rural and urban samples in 1993 and 2004 are available on request.

3 Dietary Transition in India

An Analysis Based on NSS Data, 1993–2004

Nidhi Kaicker, Vani S. Kulkarni, and
Raghav Gaiha

Rapid economic growth, urbanization, and globalization have resulted in dietary shifts in Asia, away from staples, and increasingly towards livestock and dairy products, fruits and vegetables, and fats and oil. Besides, current consumption patterns seem to be converging towards a Western diet (Pingali 2007; Popkin *et al.* 2012).[1]

These dietary changes reflect interaction of demand and supply factors.[2] The demand factors include: rapid income growth and urbanization, bringing about new dietary needs; and more generally, growing affluence and lifestyle changes. As incomes rise, exposure to the global 'urban' eating patterns increases. Recent evidence also points to greater reliance of smaller and poorer households on street food. Urban slums often mimic the branded products of fast food outlets (Pingali 2007). On the supply side, the main factors associated with the availability of food are: closer integration of global economies, severing of the link between local production and availability of food; liberalization of foreign direct investment, with a new role of multinational corporations (MNCs);[3] and a sharp reduction in freight and transportation costs (Pingali 2007).

According to recent projections, by 2020, half of the world's population will be urban and, Asia alone will account for half that population. Urban population worldwide, estimated at about 2.9 billion in 2000, is projected to reach 4.9 billion by 2030. Most of the increase will be in the cities of developing countries (UNFPA 2001).

Growing affluence and urbanization bring in their wake not just lifestyle changes with implications for food demand, but also supply side effects. Large urban markets favour supermarket chains that impact the entire food supply chain. Vertically integrated food supply chain that links input suppliers, producers, processors, distributors, and retailers becomes essential for meeting the changing demand requirements. Expansion of agricultural trade and advances in transportation and communications contribute towards convergence of diets. Trade liberalization, for example, facilitates establishment of global supermarket chains and fast food outlets, and thus contributes to the diffusion of homogenous foods and a global diet in the Asian market (Pingali 2007).

THE INDIAN EXPERIENCE

India is currently undergoing a rapid economic and demographic transformation. Since 1980, average living standards have experienced a sustained and rapid rise. The gross domestic product (GDP) per capita has risen by 230 per cent; a trend rate of 4 per cent annually. Life expectancy has risen from 54 years to 69 years, while the (crude) birth rate has fallen from 34 to 22 per thousand between 1980 and 2008. Rapid economic growth has been accompanied by rising urbanization. Between 1980 and 2000, the share of the urban population rose from 23 to 28 per cent. By 2030, it is likely to be as high as 41 per cent.

The growth momentum was accelerated by wide ranging domestic and external liberalization of the Indian economy in the last two decades. A key feature of the economic transformation has been the change in the nature of the Indian diet—a shift away from cereals and towards vanaspati oil, eggs, meat, fish and poultry, fruits and vegetables—but with rural-urban variation.

Some of the underlying factors of this dietary transition include expansion of the middle class, higher female participation, the emergence of nuclear two-income families, a sharp age divide in food preferences (with younger age groups more susceptible to new foods advertised in the media), and a rapid growth of supermarkets and fast-food outlets.[4]

With greater urbanization, demographic changes, increased participation of females in the workforce, and a growing middle class, there has been an increasingly greater prevalence of eating out as well as consumption of snacks, beverages, and pre-cooked meals. Moreover, even the more deprived sections have not been left out of these changes in dietary patterns. The analysis in Chapter 4 reveals interesting results on the phenomenon of eating out. It is a feature not just of metros and urban areas, but also of urban slums and rural areas, although the prevalence is larger in the former category. Further, it is a feature not just of the affluent sections, but also of the poor and other deprived sections. However, the (relatively) affluent are more likely to eat out and also spend greater amounts. While eating out was slightly more common in joint families than among nuclear families, among those who ate out, more than half belonged to nuclear families. The likelihood of households eating out increases with the number of adults (both males and females) in paid employment.

The health implications of the dietary transition are unclear. A more varied and nutritionally balanced diet and higher levels of food hygiene are associated with better health. But there is a trade-off as more energy-dense foods are linked to higher incidence of diet-related non-communicable diseases (NCDs) such as diabetes, coronary heart disease, and certain types of cancer.[5] Although India lags behind other developing countries in the epidemiological transition—decline in infectious disease mortality compensated for increasingly by higher mortality from chronic degenerative NCDs—there is some evidence of this transition taking place. Estimated deaths from NCDs are projected to rise from 3.78 million in 1990 (40.46 per cent of all deaths) to 7.63 million in 2020 (66.70 per cent of all deaths). Worse, about a quarter of the deaths occurred in the 35 to 64 age group in urban areas (Kulkarni and Gaiha 2010).[6]

In a comprehensive study, Mahal *et al.* (2009) demonstrate that NCDs constitute a major economic burden in India. They report high levels of out-of-pocket spending by households with members suffering from NCDs, limited levels of insurance coverage (including subsidized public services), and the income losses that befall affected households.

Associated with these costs are risks of catastrophic spending and impoverishment, and, of course, macro impacts.[7]

The focus of this chapter is on the nutritional implications of the dietary transition sketched earlier. As this has not been examined so far, our analysis is the first of its kind in a demand theory framework.

If we go by the per capita calorie norms of 2,100 for urban areas and 2,400 for the rural, the proportion of calorie deficient population rose over the period 1993–2004, from about 58 per cent to about 64 per cent in urban areas, from about 71 per cent to about 80 per cent in rural areas, and from about 68 per cent to about 76 per cent at the all-India level. The decline in mean calorie intake from 2,156 in 1993 to 2,047 in 2004 for rural India and from 2,074 in 1993 to 2,021 in 2004 for urban India is attributed to the decline in calorie intake from cereals, which was only partially offset by the increase in calorie intake from vanaspati oil and eggs (in both rural and urban areas), and milk (only in urban areas).

As noted earlier, in an influential contribution, Deaton and Dréze (2009)[8] offer the conjecture that much of the reduction in calorie intake reflects lower calorie 'requirements' due to lifestyle changes (more sedentary lifestyles), less strenuous activities, and improvements in the social epidemiology of disease. They are somewhat dismissive of the role of relative food prices in causing dietary changes.[9] Arguably, the food price index constructed by them is much too aggregate to address this issue.

As people demand and consume food commodities, it is important to understand better the nature of dietary changes and the factors underlying them before offering a definitive verdict on why under-nutrition worsened, if at all. The present study aims to do this in a demand theory framework that allows for not just price and income/expenditure effects, but also encompasses the role of changing lifestyles and activity patterns over time. The period chosen for this analysis is 1993–2004.

The scheme is as follows. A review of changes in the diets in rural and urban samples of the National Sample Survey (NSS) data over the period 1993–2004 is carried out in this chapter. It discusses the construction of a Food Diversity Index (FDI), and anayses its determinants.[10] The methodology used for estimation of demand functions for eight commodities and regression results are discussed in the Annexure.

The effect of FDI on calorie intake is analysed using instrumental variable (IV) estimation. This raises doubts about a common presumption that food diversity and quality of diet go together (EIU 2012). The concluding pages offer observations from a broad policy perspective.

CHANGES IN DIETS

A few salient features of changes in diet composition are discussed below. Table 3.1 shows the daily per capita food intake (in grams) for both rural and urban India in 1993 and 2004. The data were taken from the 50th and 61st rounds of the NSS (corresponding to 1993–4 and 2004–5, respectively).

Let us first examine the changes in food consumed in rural India. There was a reduction of about 10 per cent in cereal consumption, a reduction of 6 per cent in sugar consumption, and a reduction of about 1 per cent in the consumption of milk. Pulses recorded an implausibly sharp drop of about 45 per cent. By contrast, intake of vanaspati oil rose by about 31 per cent. Intake of vegetables and meat rose, but only slightly. Consumption of fruits, and eggs, on the other hand, rose sharply. Reduction in cereal intake was lower in urban India (about 7 per cent). As in the rural samples, pulses recorded a somewhat drastic reduction of about 37 per cent. Sugar recorded a reduction of about 10 per cent. The consumption of milk increased in urban areas (by 4 per cent). While meat, fruits, milk, and vegetables recorded small increases, eggs and vanaspati oil recorded moderately higher intakes.

There are considerable variations in the consumption of these commodities by the median and 75th percentile households. The declines in consumption of cereals for the median and 75th percentile households were not so dissimilar (~10 per cent in rural and ~8 per cent in urban areas). The decline was more for the 75th percentile households than the median households in case of sugar. By contrast, while the consumption of pulses declined by 54 per cent for the median households in rural areas, the decline was only 9 per cent for the 75th percentile households. In urban areas, the decline was almost equal (~35 per cent). The consumption of Vanaspati oil, fruits, and vegetable increased in both rural and urban areas, with little or no variation between the median and the 75th percentile households, as well as for eggs, but with a greater variation.

TABLE 3.1 Daily Per Capita Consumption of Food Commodities (grams), 1993 and 2004

Year	Cereals	Milk Products Ghee/Butter	Vanaspati Oil	Sugar	Eggs	Meat/Fish/ Poultry	Pulses/Nuts/ Dry Fruits	Fruits	Vegetables
Rural India									
1993									
Median	456.6	96.5	12.1	24.7	1.2	10.1	368.7	13.5	161.7
75th percentile	476.0	144.6	14.5	31.0	1.5	12.8	445.1	19.5	177
Total	446.8	113.4	12.4	26.2	1.2	10.5	368.6	16.4	158
2004									
Median	412.4	108.0	16.0	24.2	1.8	9.8	170.3	17.1	170.8
75th percentile	425.7	152.0	19.1	29.8	2.6	14.1	404.6	24.0	189.8
Total	404	111.7	16.2	24.7	1.9	11.3	203.4	19.6	167.7
Urban India									
1993									
Median	366.3	132.9	18.7	33.0	2.5	13.0	459.5	26.3	164.1
75th percentile	362.5	181.3	22.2	38.5	3.3	15.5	631.7	36.4	185.7
Total	354.7	143	18.7	32.4	2.9	13.9	520.8	32.4	167.4
2004									
Median	336.0	149.4	23.1	30.4	3.2	12.7	302.4	30.3	178.7
75th percentile	332.4	193.0	26.9	33.8	4.5	17.2	407.5	43.2	204.2
Total	331.4	149	22.1	29	3.3	14.1	327	33.1	182.4

Source: Computed from 50th and 61st rounds of the NSS, corresponding to 1993–4 and 2004–5.

In both rural and urban areas, the increase in consumption of milk for the median households (~12 per cent) was double that of the 75th percentile households (~6 per cent). While the consumption of meat decreased for the median households, there was an increase for the 75th percentile households, in both rural and urban areas. It is noteworthy that the pattern of dietary change is different for low and higher expenditure classes.

Thus food composition/diet changed considerably in both rural and urban areas over the period 1993–2004. While consumption of cereals, sugar, and pulses has declined, there has been an increase in the consumption of high-value commodities such as vanaspati oil, eggs, fruits, and vegetables, and to some extent, of meat as well. As these changes are linked to intakes of calories, proteins and fats with varying importance, an investigation of how food consumption patterns changed in response to changes in income and relative prices is necessary.

Food Diversity Index

To assess diversity in food consumption, one approach is to count the number of food items consumed by a household. As this does not allow for their relative importance in food expenditure, we have followed a different approach which relies on their shares in food expenditure, with 2004 prices as weights. To capture diversification in diets, that is, a move from a cereal dominated diet to more variety in it, we construct a Food Diversity Index (FDI). The FDI is calculated as the sum of squares of the shares of the various food items in the consumption basket. Algebraically,

$$FDI_{it} = \sum_{j=1}^{5} S_{jit}^{2} \tag{1}$$

where FDI_{it} is the food diversity index for household i at time period t, and S_{jit} is the share of jth commodity in the food consumption basket. This is similar to the Herfindahl index used to measure the competitiveness of an industry. In percentages, the value of this index lies between 0 and 100. High value of the index implies a monopolistic industry (or, in our case, a more concentrated food basket), and low value implies nearly perfectly competitive industry (in our case, a more diverse food basket). We use five food groups to construct the FDI:

(i) cereals and pulses; (ii) milk, milk products, eggs, and meats; (iii) oil; (iv) sugar; and (iv) fruits and vegetables. We consider a less disaggregated classification of food commodities than used before, but there is no more than a slight loss of information. Tables 3.2 and 3.3 give the FDI indices at the all-India level for 1993 and 2004, and the shares of food commodities by per capita expenditure deciles.

Both in 1993 and 2004, these indices fall across expenditure deciles. In 1993, the FDI index fell from 49.38 per cent in the first decile to 32.46 per cent in the 10th decile, implying greater diversification among the more affluent. In 2004, the index was smaller among the first decile (40.50 per cent), as compared with the value in 1993, suggest-

TABLE 3.2 Food Diversification in India, 1993–4

1993–4 All-India	FDI	Share of Cereals and Pulses (%)	Share of Meat, Milk, and Eggs (%)	Share of Fruits and Veg (%)	Share of Oil (%)	Share of Sugar (%)
10th percentile	49.38	65	10	14	8	4
25th percentile	43.54	59	14	14	8	5
50th percentile	38.23	53	20	15	8	5
75th percentile	34.01	44	26	16	8	6
90th percentile	32.46	37	30	18	9	6

Source: Authors' calculations from the 50th round of the NSS. These percentiles are in ascending order of per capita expenditure.

TABLE 3.3 Food Diversification in India, 2004–5

2004–5 All-India	FDI	Share of Cereals and Pulses (%)	Share of Meat, Milk, and Eggs (%)	Share of Fruits and Veg (%)	Share of Oil (%)	Share of Sugar (%)
10th percentile	40.50	56	12	18	10	4
25th percentile	36.79	52	16	17	10	5
50th percentile	33.94	47	22	17	10	4
75th percentile	31.71	40	28	18	9	5
90th percentile	31.49	35	32	20	9	4

Source: Authors' calculations from the 61st round of the NSS. These percentiles are in ascending order of per capita expenditure.

ing greater diversification even among the poorest. The corresponding value for the 10th decile was, however, only slightly lower than in 1993 (31.49 per cent as compared with 32.46 per cent). This comparison suggests that the diversification among the affluent was much slower than among the poorest.

If we go by the shares of food commodities in the food expenditure, share of cereals and pulses fell rapidly from 65 per cent among the poorest to 37 per cent among the most affluent in 1993; that of milk was much higher among the latter (30 per cent as compared with 10 per cent); and the share of fruits was slightly higher (18 per cent as compared with 14 per cent). The shares of oil and sugar were only slightly higher.[11]

Let us now examine the dietary changes in rural India during 1993–2004, as shown in Tables 3.4 and 3.5. Across expenditure deciles, there is a sharp reduction in the FDI, from 50.81 per cent among the poorest to 33.88 per cent among the most affluent, implying considerably greater diversification among the latter. In 2004, the poorest had diversified considerably, while the affluent had diversified much less. The shares of food expenditure in 1993 revealed a pattern similar to that at the all-India level: rapid reduction in shares of cereals and pulses, a rapid rise in that of meat, milk, and eggs, and slightly higher shares of vegetables, oil, and sugar. A pattern similar to 1993 is discernible for 2004, except that shares of vegetables, oil, and sugar were slightly lower among the affluent compared to the poorest. Also, relative to 1993, shares of cereals among the poorest

TABLE 3.4 Food Diversification in Rural India, 1993–4

1993–4 Rural	FDI	Share of Cereals and Pulses (%)	Share of Meat, Milk, and Eggs (%)	Share of Fruits and Vegetables (%)	Share of Oil (%)	Share of Sugar (%)
10th percentile	50.81	66	8	14	7	4
25th percentile	44.74	61	13	14	8	5
50th percentile	40.36	55	18	14	8	5
75th percentile	36.57	48	24	15	8	5
90th percentile	33.88	41	29	16	8	6

Source: Authors' calculations from the 50th round of the NSS. These percentiles are in ascending order of per capita expenditure.

TABLE 3.5 Food Diversification in Rural India, 2004–5

2004–5 Rural	FDI	Share of Cereals & Pulses (%)	Share of Meat, Milk, & Eggs (%)	Share of Fruits & Veg (%)	Share of Oil (%)	Share of Sugar (%)
10th percentile	41.03	57	11	18	10	4
25th percentile	37.18	53	15	17	10	5
50th percentile	34.51	48	20	17	10	5
75th percentile	32.71	43	25	17	9	5
90th percentile	31.65	38	31	17	9	5

Source: Authors' calculations from the 61st round of the NSS. These percentiles are in ascending order of per capita expenditure.

were considerably lower in 2004, but only slightly among the affluent; shares of meat and milk were slightly higher among both groups; shares of fruits and vegetables rose among the poorest moderately, but only slightly among the affluent; and there were negligible changes in the shares of oil and sugar.

Tables 3.6 and 3.7 throw light on food diversification in urban India in 1993–2004. If we go by the values of the FDI in urban India in 1993, a somewhat surprising finding is that food diversification was moderately greater among the affluent relative to the poorest. In 2004, the poorest diversified more than moderately, while the affluent recorded lower diversification. Shares of cereals were a little over

TABLE 3.6 Food Diversification in Urban India, 1993–4

1993–4 Urban	FDI	Share of Cereals and Pulses (%)	Share of Meat, Milk, and Eggs (%)	Share of Fruits and Veg (%)	Share of Oil (%)	Share of Sugar (%)
10th percentile	40.21	56	15	15	9	5
25th percentile	36.43	51	19	15	9	5
50th percentile	32.90	42	25	17	9	6
75th percentile	32.63	36	29	20	9	5
90th percentile	36.33	29	32	26	9	5

Source: Authors' calculations from the 50th round of the NSS. These percentiles are in ascending order of per capita expenditure.

TABLE 3.7 Food Diversification in Urban India, 2004–5

2004–5 Urban	FDI	Share of Cereals and Pulses (%)	Share of Meat, Milk, and Eggs (%)	Share of Fruits and Veg (%)	Share of Oil (%)	Share of Sugar (%)
10th percentile	34.74	47	20	19	9	5
25th percentile	32.78	43	25	19	8	5
50th percentile	31.79	40	29	18	8	5
75th percentile	32.96	35	32	21	7	4
90th percentile	34.22	31	35	23	7	4

Source: Authors' calculations from the 61st round of the NSS. These percentiles are in ascending order of per capita expenditure.

a half of that among the poorest in 1993. In 2004, while the share among the poorest was lower, it rose slightly among the affluent. Share of meat and milk was higher among the poorest, but rose moderately among the affluent. Share of fruits and vegetables was higher among the poorest, but fell among the affluent, as also shares of oil and sugar albeit slightly.

A graphical representation of variation in FDI by per capita expenditure is given in Figure 3.1. Diets were more diversified at higher expenditure levels. Besides, diet diversification was greater in 2004 than in 1993. However, among households below the median monthly per capita expenditure (MPCE), diet diversification was much faster over the period 1993–2004.

METHODOLOGY

We report our findings on changing dietary patterns of Indian households based on an analysis of the 1993 and 2004 household surveys conducted by the NSS.[12] Estimation at the household level is preferred as there is greater variation in expenditure levels than found in grouped data. An Instrumental Variables estimation is used. First, a reduced form demand relation is used in which the dependent variable is the FDI, as defined earlier, and the right side/explanatory variables include prices of food commodities, income, household characteristics, and the general environment (lifestyle changes, healthier environment).[13]

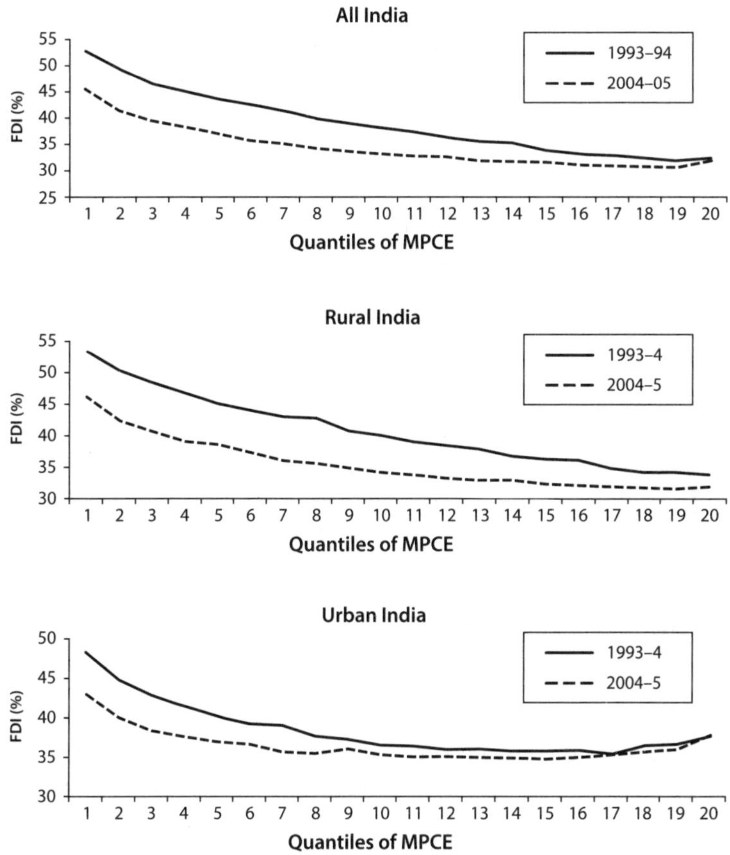

FIGURE **3.1** Food Diversity Index at Various Levels of MPCE
Source: Authors' calculations based on NSS (50th and 61st rounds).

$$\text{FDI}_{it} = \alpha + \boldsymbol{P}_{jt}\boldsymbol{\beta} + \gamma E_{it} + \boldsymbol{X}_{it}\boldsymbol{\delta} + \partial CD_{it} + \lambda_1 D1_t + \theta RD1 + \vartheta RD2 + \varepsilon_{it} \quad (2)$$

Where the dependent variable is the food diversity index for *ith* household in time *t*, $\boldsymbol{P}_{jt}$ is a vector of food prices (for selected commodity groups) computed from the NSS at the village level (*j*) and time *t*; E_{it} is household per capita expenditure of *ith* household in time *t*; $\boldsymbol{X}_{jt}$ is a vector of household characteristics (for example number of adult males, females, household size, whether adult males and females possessed middle or higher level of education) and a few others specified as dummy variables (caste and education); $D1_t$ is a dummy variable that takes the value 1 for 2004 and 0 otherwise (to allow for changes in factors other than food prices and expenditure over time); two regional dummies, *RD*1 and *RD*2, denoting BIMARU (Bihar, Madhya Pradesh, Rajasthan, and Uttar Pradesh) and coastal states, respectively, and whether a household belongs to a middle class or not; CD_{it} based on whether it owns consumer durables (for example, a TV), and ε_{it} is the error term.[14] As dietary transition is closely linked to the emergence of the middle class (Deolalikar 2010; Pingali 2007; Popkin *et al.* 2012), the latter serves as an instrument for the food diversity equation. The regional dummies for BIMARU and coastal states are justified on the grounds that the first subset is among the poorest while the latter are among the more prosperous. An innovative feature of this specification is that both price and expenditure variables are interacted with time to allow for changes in their coefficients over time.

In the second stage, calories consumed per capita per day, $Calories_{it}$, are regressed on all exogenous variables in the reduced form except the instrument, CD_{it}, as shown below:

$$\text{Calories}_{it} = \alpha + \boldsymbol{P}_{jt}\boldsymbol{\beta} + \gamma E_{it} + \boldsymbol{X}_{it}\boldsymbol{\delta} + \pi \widehat{FD}_{it} + \lambda_1 D1_t + \theta RD1 + \vartheta RD2 + u_{it} \quad (3)$$

As may be noted, all right side variables are the same as in equation 2 except that the instrument is omitted while an instrumented value of FDI is inserted, $\widehat{FDI}_{it}$ Standard errors are corrected for heteroscedasticity.

RESULTS

The robust regression results are discussed below (Tables 3.8 and 3.9).[15]

FDI and cereal prices are negatively related. The higher the cereal price, the lower is food diversification, suggesting lower consumption of cereals and their substitution by cheaper sources of calories. This effect weakens with time, as reflected in a positive coefficient of cereal price with time. In fact, it largely offsets the negative effect of cereal price. Ratio of cereal price to that of meat and milk has a negative coefficient. Since cereal price is given, a higher ratio implies a fall in the price of meat and milk, and a higher demand for these products. Interaction of this price ratio with time partly weakens this effect, but the two together imply greater diversification. The second ratio has

TABLE 3.8 Instrumental Variables Regression Results—First Stage

Dependent Variable: Food Diversity Index	Number of Obs. = 221832 F(19, 221812) = 2560.91 Prob>F = 0.0000		
	Coefficient		
Time Dummy (1993=0, 2004=1)	−1.55	(−11.15)	***
Price of Cereals and Pulses	−1.14	(−26.52)	***
Interaction (Price of Cereals and Pulses Time Dummy)*	1.13	(24.82)	***
Price Ratio of Cereals and Pulses to Milk and Milk Products	−5.49	(−52.46)	***
Interaction (Price Ratio of Cereals and Pulses to Milk and Milk Products Time Dummy)*	2.40	(18.81)	***
Price Ratio of Cereals and Pulses *to* Vanaspati Oil	45.51	(33.84)	***
Interaction (Price Ratio of Cereals and Pulses to Vanaspati Oil Time Dummy)*	−46.47	(−29.39)	***
MPCE at 2004 Prices	0.00	(−4.29)	***
Interaction (MPCE at 2004 prices Time Dummy)*	0.00	(4.16)	***
Household Size	0.39	(44.03)	***
Proportion of Adults in the household	−0.05	(−0.63)	**
Education Dummy Males (Above Middle education =1)	−1.39	(−34.62)	***
Education Dummy Females (Above Middle education =1)	−1.34	(−35.71)	***
Caste Dummy (ST =1, Ref Category = SC)	0.06	(0.8)	**
Caste Dummy (Others =1, Ref Category = SC)	−0.82	(−12.8)	***
Sector Dummy (Urban = 1)	−1.70	(−43.11)	***
State Dummy (Bimaru = 1)	−0.64	(−12.65)	***
State Dummy (Coastal States = 1)	−0.44	(−10.88)	***
Ownership of consumer durables (Instrument)	−4.11	(−61.57)	***
Constant	39.15	(264.41)	

Source: Authors' calculations based on NSS (50th and 61st rounds).

Note: ***, **, and * refer to 1 per cent, 5 per cent, and 10 per cent significance levels, respectively.

cereal price relative to vanaspati oil. This has a positive coefficient, but its interaction with time yields a negative coefficient that more than offsets the positive effect, implying greater demand for vanaspati oil and diversification of diet.[16]

Per capita expenditure lowers the FDI, as emphasized in the extant literature, but the effect is small. This is enhanced by the positive coefficient of the interaction term.

Household characteristics also influence diets: the larger the household size, the lower is the food diversification; if adult males and females possess middle or higher level of education, it is associated with greater food diversity; and 'others' (as a residual caste group) exhibit greater diversity relative to the omitted group of SCs.

Location matters too. After accounting for all other effects, those residing in urban areas have more diversified diets. Those living in BIMARU states—still among the poorest states in India—show greater food diversity, as also those in coastal states, relative to the remaining. This is an important finding, confirming that dietary transformation is not confined to the affluent regions, and is also occurring among the poorest.

The identifying variable, whether a household belongs to the middle class, has a negative coefficient, confirming the relevance of the instrument. The joint significance of all exogenous variables is corroborated by the F-statistic.

EFFECT OF FDI ON CALORIE INTAKE

The effect of time requires elaboration. The time dummy (1 for 2004 and 0 otherwise) has a significant negative coefficient, implying that lifestyle changes (for example sedentary lifestyles, less strenuous activity patterns, nuclearization of families, preference for variety in food) have led to dietary diversification. In addition, the effect of time is mediated through changes in price and expenditure effects.

Our results in Table 3.9 focus on the effects of dietary diversification on calorie intake. While hints exist in the extant literature (Pingali 2007; Popkin *et al.* 2012; Shetty 2002), precise estimates of the effect of dietary diversification on calorie intake are lacking.

There is robust confirmation of the positive effect of the (instrumented) FDI on calorie intake. Since a higher value of FDI indicates

TABLE 3.9 Instrumental Variables Regression Results—Second Stage

Dependent Variable: Calorie Intake	Number of Obs. = 221832 F(19, 221812) = 818.73 Prob>F = 0.0000		
	Coefficient		
Predicted value of Food Diversity Index from 1st Stage	21.48	(4.49)	***
Time Dummy (1993=0, 2004=1)	−72.84	(−2.08)	**
Price of Cereals and Pulses	−37.64	(−3.49)	***
Interaction (Price of Cereals and Pulses Time Dummy)*	−11.27	(−0.67)	**
Price Ratio of Cereals and Pulses to Milk and Milk Products	397.79	(12.08)	***
Interaction (Price Ratio of Cereals and Pulses to Milk and Milk Products Time Dummy)*	−299.43	(−7.88)	***
Price Ratio of Cereals and Pulses to Vanaspati Oil	390.48	(1.33)	**
Interaction (Price Ratio of Cereals and Pulses to Vanaspati Oil Time Dummy)*	2198.28	(2.79)	***
MPCE at 2004 Prices	0.24	(4.14)	***
Interaction (MPCE at 2004 prices Time Dummy)*	−0.02	(−0.3)	**
Household Size	−56.99	(−24.14)	***
Proportion of Adults in the household	732.93	(44.2)	***
Education Dummy Males (Above Middle education =1)	146.96	(14.38)	***
Education Dummy Females (Above Middle education =1)	47.96	(5.32)	***
Caste Dummy (ST =1, Ref Category = SC)	−69.60	(−4.42)	***
Caste Dummy (Others =1, Ref Category = SC)	51.89	(3.94)	***
Sector Dummy (Urban = 1)	−141.78	(−12.38)	***
State Dummy (Bimaru = 1)	59.90	(6.35)	***
State Dummy (Coastal States = 1)	−207.32	(−23.55)	***
Constant	1123.26	(5.72)	

Source: Authors' calculations based on NSS (50th and 61st rounds).

*Note:****, **, and * refer to 1 per cent, 5 per cent, and 10 per cent significance levels, respectively.

concentration of consumers on a few items (cereals are the single largest source of calories), it implies that calorie intake is higher. Or the greater the diversification (implied by a lower value of FDI), the lower is the calorie intake. This is an aspect that has not been sufficiently emphasized, or simply glossed over in recent studies (Deaton and Dréze 2009).

As the link between calorie intake and dietary diversification is the principal focus of this chapter, our comments on the remaining results are brief.[17]

Food price effects are significant. Cereal price lowers calorie intake and this effect is reinforced by the interaction with time. Cereal price relative to meat and milk increases calorie intake (through substitution of energy from fats); but this effect is substantially weakened by interaction of this price with time. Cereal price relative to oil has a positive but non-significant effect. The interaction term, however, has a positive and significant coefficient, implying that over time oil has contributed to greater calorie intake (for example, preference for fried foods, potato chips, etc.). Expenditure has a positive effect on calories, but there is a slight weakening over time. Household size has a significant negative coefficient, implying a lower calorie intake. This is not surprising in view of the positive coefficient of proportion of adults. So, if the proportion of adults is fixed, larger households imply larger number of children and lower calorie demand. More educated adult male and female members are associated with greater calorie intake. If this has to be reconciled with the result on dietary diversification in Table 3.8, it is plausible that while education helps diversify diets, it also enables more balanced or healthier diets. STs consume lower calories, while 'others' consume more relative to SCs. Urban areas exhibit a significant reduction in calorie intake relative to rural areas, after accounting for all other effects in this equation. BIMARU states consume more calories, while coastal states consume fewer calories than other states. Whether BIMARU states are diversifying, with higher calories, needs further investigation.

Over and above these effects, lifestyle changes associated with time (more sedentary lifestyles, less strenuous activity patterns, improvements in the epidemiology of infectious disease environment) contributed to lower calorie 'requirements', and thus intake. But as noted above, time also influenced calorie intake through changes in price and expenditure effects.

The null of under-identification is rejected by the Kleinberger-Paap rk LM statistic, and the equation is just identified. The weak instrument null is also rejected by the Kleinberger-Paap rk Wald F statistic. Together with the relevance of the instrument, it is validated.

In sum, food prices, urbanization, expansion of the middle class, and lifestyle changes contributed to dietary diversification, which in turn resulted in lower calorie intake.[18]

***

Recent studies show that despite rising incomes in India, there has been a sustained decline in per capita calorie intake over the period 1983–2004, primarily due to lower calorie 'requirements'. The reduction in calorie requirements is attributed mainly to better health environment and less strenuous activity levels. Departing from this focus, but encompassing it in an alternative demand theory based explanation of dietary changes, the present study analysed first the factors associated with dietary diversification, and then in the second stage the effect of dietary diversification on calorie intake. Dietary diversification is associated with food prices, income/expenditure, household characteristics (especially whether it belongs to the middle class) and its location, and time related changes transmitted through prices and expenditure, and residually through lifestyle, activity patterns, and improvements in the epidemiology of disease environment. The more important result, however, is the lowering of calorie intake as a result of dietary diversification, controlling for the effects of food prices, expenditure, household characteristics (other than middle class affiliation), urban location, and time related changes. The latter adds an important dimension to food and health policies.

Supermarkets are increasingly driving the food policy agenda. While they offer greater consumer choice and lower prices, they consolidate the supply chain to only a few producers who are increasingly responsible for compliance with the cost, quality, and safety standards. The state, therefore, has to play a proactive role in laying down food safety standards and in ensuring their compliance.

The health implications of the changes in dietary patterns are not clear cut. There is a trade-off—while a nutritionally balanced diet is associated with better health, energy dense foods are responsible for higher prevalence of NCDs such as heart disease, cancer, and diabetes. Since there are signs of an epidemiological transition in India—higher mortality from these diseases compensating for decline in mortality from infectious diseases—enhancing awareness of healthy diets is important from a policy perspective. As consumer preferences for flavour, packaging, and variety evolve in complex ways in a context of rapidly integrating food markets, a careful scrutiny of measures (labelling of food quality, consumer awareness campaigns through the media and other channels) may help understand better how to influence food choices.

In sum, not just food availability, but also how a healthy diet could be promoted raise serious policy concerns.

ANNEXURE

Demand Functions for Food Commodities

As demand for nutrients in general, and for calories in particular, are derived from demands for different food commodities, we summarize here food commodity demand functions. In addition, we examine determinants of an alternative FDI (but not as informative as the FDI based on the Herfindahl index).

We will discuss the results obtained from pooled rural and urban samples for 1993 and 2004, given in Table 3A.1.

The demand for each of the commodities analysed is inversely related to its own price, consistent with demand theory. The magnitude of elasticity (in absolute terms), however, varies. While the demand for cereals, meat, and vegetables is highly responsive to price change, the responsiveness of the demand for fruits and pulses is moderate, and that of vanaspati oil and eggs is small. An increase in the price of milk leads to a negligible reduction in its demand—a case of highly inelastic demand.

While there are significant own price effects, there have been shifts in these effects between 1993 and 2004.[19] The price effect has become stronger for cereals, milk, meat, pulses, and vegetables. The shift in the price effect is negative for vanaspati oil. Thus, the price effects in most cases vary with time. Arguably, these variations reflect changing food preferences over time—preferences for taste and variety.

TABLE 3A.1 Elasticities (based on robust regression results for cereals and tobit estimations for other commodities)

	(1) Cereals	(2) Milk/Milk Products/ Ghee/Butter	(3) Vanaspati Oil	(4) Eggs	(5) Meat/ Poultry/ Fish	(6) Pulses/ Nuts/Others	(7) Fruits	(8) Vegetables	(9) Food Diversity
Time Dummy (0=1993, 1=2004)	−0.072 (−29.68) ***	−0.034 (−26.07) ***	0.087 (9.68) ***	0.043 (14.48) ***	0.003 (0.71) –	−0.041 (−20.9) ***	0.025 (11.11) ***	0.040 (12.02) ***	0.023 (7.83) ***
Price	−0.300 (−55.96) ***	−0.005 (−3.65) ***	−0.037 (−1.96) *	−0.022 (−10.5) ***	−0.305 (−41.0) ***	−0.126 (−38.0) ***	−0.103 (−27.49) ***	−0.311 (−45.2) ***	−0.370 (−90.34) ***
Time Dummy X Price	0.085 (24.85) ***	0.002 (2.57) **	−0.050 (−3.73) ***	0.002 (0.6) –	0.091 (16.65) ***	0.060 (23.22) ***	−0.004 (−1.48) –	0.049 (10.27) ***	−0.045 (−16.65) ***
Per Capita Expenditure (MPCE)	0.120 (192.32) ***	0.129 (257.38) ***	0.084 (99.91) ***	0.080 (59.02) ***	0.066 (52.32) ***	0.023 (23.67) ***	0.105 (127.73) ***	0.071 (84.02) ***	−0.283 (−235.0) ***
Square of MPCE	−0.043 (−1246) ***	−0.002 (−124.0) ***	−0.001 (−45.7) ***	−0.003 (−33.64) ***	−0.003 (−26.8) ***	0.000 (−14.3) ***	−0.002 (−63.99) ***	−0.001 (−42.1) ***	0.095 (841.2) ***
Household Size	0.002 (1.61) –	0.051 (22.18) ***	−0.029 (−12.8) ***	−0.004 (−1.46) –	0.036 (14.72) ***	−0.048 (−22.4) ***	0.004 (1.94) *	−0.105 (−46.9) ***	0.046 (18.86) ***

(continued)

TABLE 3A.1 Continued

	(1) Cereals	(2) Milk/Milk Products/ Ghee/Butter	(3) Vanaspati Oil	(4) Eggs	(5) Meat/ Poultry/ Fish	(6) Pulses/ Nuts/Others	(7) Fruits	(8) Vegetables	(9) Food Diversity
Proportion of Adults in the Household	0.179 (101.11) ★★★	0.110 (35.45) ★★★	0.133 (41.72) ★★★	0.001 (0.25) –	−0.005 (−1.44) –	0.031 (10.51) ★★★	0.031 (9.68) ★★★	0.178 (56.51) ★★★	0.036 (9.77) ★★★
Caste Dummy (ST)	0.000 (0.03) –	0.009 (9.07) ★★★	0.009 (10.17) ★★★	−0.003 (−3.26) ★★★	−0.006 (−6.59) ★★★	0.000 (−0.12) –	0.001 (0.92) –	0.005 (6.07) ★★★	−0.005 (−5.94) ★★★
Caste Dummy (Others)	−0.015 (−9.91) ★★★	0.183 (58.62) ★★★	0.057 (20.81) ★★★	−0.008 (−2.16) ★★	−0.045 (−15.9) ★★★	−0.001 (−0.39) –	0.059 (20.13) ★★★	0.043 (15.89) ★★★	−0.132 (−42.89) ★★★
Sector Dummy (0=rural, 1=urban)	−0.049 (−100) ★★★	−0.005 (−7.15) ★★★	0.011 (16.02) ★★★	0.007 (7.6) ★★★	−0.002 (−2.65) ★★★	0.004 (6.51) ★★★	0.017 (25.97) ★★★	0.006 (8.43) ★★★	−0.025 (−26.92) ★★★

Source: Authors' calculations based on NSS (50th and 61st rounds).

Notes: The dependent variable is the daily per capita consumption of the commodity (in grams) for columns (1) to (8). The dependent variable in column (9) is the FDI.

The 'Price' variable refers to the price index of commodity in columns (1) to (8). In column (9), the price refers to the ratio of prices of cereals and pulses to the prices of all other commodities, weighted **by prices** of these commodities in 2004.

The reference category for the Caste Dummy is the *Scheduled Castes*.

State Dummies have been omitted in the above table and shall be available on request.

★★★, ★★, and ★ refer to significance at the 1 per cent, 5 per cent, and 10 per cent level of significance, respectively.

For each of the commodities, the demand increases as the monthly per capita expenditure (a proxy for income) goes up. However, at higher levels of per capita expenditure, there is a slight decline in all cases. Although the expenditure elasticity is positive, there is considerable variation in its magnitude among the commodities—the demand is highly responsive to income in case of eggs, meat, and fruits, moderately responsive in case of milk and pulses, and least responsive in case of vegetables and vanaspati oil. The expenditure elasticity is the smallest for cereals.

Household characteristics, such as size, proportion of adults, and caste affiliation have significant impacts on the demand for various food commodities. As household size increases, the demand for milk and meat increases, and for vegetables, pulses, and vanaspati oil decreases. With higher proportion of adults in a household, the demand for all commodities goes up, except eggs and meat, where there is no impact. In the case of vegetables, pulses, and vanaspati oil, where the household size has a negative impact but the proportion of adults in a household has a positive impact, the explanation lies partly in lower demand for these commodities from children, and partly in the economies of scale arising out of cooking in a household.

The links between caste affiliation and demand for food commodities are interesting. In comparison to SCs, 'others' demanded larger amounts of milk, vanaspati oil, fruits, and vegetables, and lower amounts of meat and cereals. This may in part reflect cultural differences among these categories.

Urbanization has a significant impact on the demand for various food commodities, although the elasticity is small. It has a positive impact on the demand for vanaspati oil, eggs, pulses, fruits, and vegetables, and a negative impact on the demand for cereals, milk, and meat. Thus, there are significant differences between urban-rural samples, pointing to urban lifestyles driving dietary changes (fatty and starchy foods).

After accounting for all other effects, there is a significant difference in the demand for these commodities between 1993 and 2004 (as captured by the time dummy). There is a higher demand for vanaspati oil, eggs, fruits, and vegetables in 2004 as compared to 1993, and a lower demand for cereals, milk, and pulses.

Dietary patterns have evolved over time as a result of less strenuous activity patterns, and more sedentary lifestyles in both rural and urban areas. As noted by Deaton and Dréze (2009), and corroborated by our analysis, these changes over time have indeed shaped dietary patterns in a decisive way. Our point of departure, however, is that this explanation is part of a demand theory based explanation, and not an alternative to it.

Food Diversity Index (FDI)

FDI is defined as a ratio of quantity of cereals and pulses consumed to that of all other food commodities, with 2004 prices as weights. So the higher is this ratio, the lower is diet diversity.

We use robust regression to estimate the impact of relative prices, incomes, and household characteristics on the FDI. The analysis is based on data pooled over both rural and urban areas, and overtime. The results are given in column 9 of Table 3A.1.

As the relative price of cereals and pulses goes up, the FDI decreases (or the dependence on cereals and pulses decreases and diet diversification occurs), consistent with demand theory. There is a negative shift in the price effect between 1993 and 2004. The elasticity of the FDI with respect to monthly per capita expenditure (a proxy for income) is negative. As income increases, a shift away from cereals and pulses towards other food items is confirmed. Both household size and proportion of adults in a household have positive effects on the demand for cereals and pulses vis-à-vis other food commodities. Consistent with the results arrived at previously—links between caste affiliation and food consumption—'others' are observed to have lower demand for cereals and pulses vis-à-vis other food items. This reflects in part cultural differences among these categories. With greater urbanization, the food diversity index is expected to fall, and the diversity to increase.

NOTES

1. This is broadly defined by high intakes of refined carbohydrates, added sugars, fats, and animal-source food. In low and middle income countries, these changes are typical of urban areas, but more recently, increasingly visible in rural areas too. Diets rich in legumes, other vegetables, and coarse grains are declining in importance in all regions and countries (Popkin *et al.* 2012).

2. As observed by Popkin *et al.* (2012), on the global level, new access to technologies (for example cheap edible oils, foods with excessive 'empty calories', modern supermarkets, and food distribution and marketing) and the regulatory environments (the World Trade Organization and freer flow of goods, services, and technologies) are changing diets.
3. Global food companies are responsible for major portions of sales of some categories of foods, such as sugar-sweetened beverages, in low and middle income countries (Popkin *et al.* 2012).
4. In a perceptive comment, Timmer (2009, 2010) addresses the following questions: impact of supermarkets on poor consumers, supply of staples, price stability, linkages with global markets, and health of consumers. While supermarkets offer greater consumer choice and lower prices, they consolidate the supply chain to only a few producers who are increasingly responsible for compliance with the cost, quality, and safety standards. Although supermarkets are increasingly driving the food policy agenda, the state has to play a proactive role in laying down food safety standards, their compliance, and in ensuring greater awareness of healthy food habits.
5. Easier access to processed foods through supermarkets is harmful as these are high in fat, added sugar, and salt. At the same time, supermarkets were instrumental in the development of ultra-heat treatment for the pasteurization of milk, giving it a longer shelf life (not requiring refrigeration) and providing a safe source of milk for all income groups. Supermarkets have also been catalysts for food safety standards. Above all, they have solved the cold chain problem and, in many cases, made available high quality produce to the urban consumer throughout the year (Popkin *et al.* 2012).
6. Mahal *et al.* (2009), Popkin *et al.* (2001), and Popkin *et al.* (2012) provide a more recent analyses of this.
7. For a rigorous and innovative analysis of the overall effect of health on income, labour productivity, savings, and population effects, see Bloom *et al.* (2009).
8. The Deaton and Dréze analysis (2009) is based on the period 1983–2004. Average calorie consumption declined by 10 per cent in rural areas between 1983 and 2004, with the proportionate decline being larger among the more affluent sections. In urban areas, there was only a slight change. The per capita consumption of proteins and other nutrients declined too, with the exception of fats whose consumption increased.
9. Popkin *et al.* (2012) is emphatic that relative food price changes matter most. If the prices of fatty foods, oils and sugar, and animal-source food go down, relative to legumes, fruits, and other vegetables, the latter items become less attractive.

10. These include cereals, milk (milk/milk products/ghee/butter), vanaspati oil, eggs, meat (meat/fish/poultry), pulses (pulses/nuts/dry fruits/others), and fruits and vegetables. Sugar was omitted as the estimates lacked precision.
11. To avoid an overload of numbers, we have reported results for selected percentiles of households in ascending order of per capita expenditure.
12. For an earlier analysis with a nationwide survey in 1994, see Jha *et al.* (2009b). This builds on Timmer (1981), and Behrman and Deolalikar (1989).
13. For a rich and comprehensive exposition of how demand functions are obtained in a neo-classical household, decision-making framework, and the shifts in these functions, see Behrman and Deolalikar (1988).
14. Various studies, more recently ADB 2010, have drawn attention to the role of the middle class in driving dietary transition. As our diagnostics show, this is a valid instrument. For an exposition of validity of instruments, see Wooldridge (2006).
15. Several other experiments were conducted, but are omitted. Details are available upon request to the authors.
16. Note that the ratio of cereal to vegetable price was dropped due to multi-collinearity.
17. As calorie demand is derived from food commodity demand, and assuming that consumers make informed food policy choices, we estimated food demand functions. The results are summarized in Annexure (in this chapter).
18. A more recent analysis (Gaiha *et al.* 2013), based on the 50th, 61st, and 66th rounds of the NSS covering 1993, 2004, and 2009, further confirms mixed nutritional effects of diet diversification. While calorie intake declined, protein and fat intake increased with diet diversification. Although opinions differ on calorie cut-offs, more than 35 per cent of rural households had calorie intake of below 1800 in 2009, pointing to pervasive calorie deprivation. Lowering of calorie intake in this context is thus not desirable. By contrast, both protein and fat intake rose in association with diet diversification. As their averages are well below the desired intakes, increases are desirable. However, given excess fat intake among moderate to large segments of the population (21 per cent of the population consumed more than 50 grams of fat), dietary shift has the potential to aggravate the risk of NCDs.
19. Results with cross-price effects in some cases lacked precision due to multi-collinearity. Hence these were omitted.

4 How Pervasive is Eating Out in India?*

Raghav Gaiha, Raghbendra Jha, and
Vani S. Kulkarni

The growth momentum during the 1980s was accelerated by wide ranging domestic and external liberalization of the Indian economy in the 1990s. A key feature of the economic transformation has been the change in the nature of the Indian diet. As the global markets integrate and communication becomes better, diet transitions are unavoidable. As shown in Chapter 3, there is a move away from inferior to superior foods, and a substitution of traditional staples by primary food products that are more prevalent in western diets. These shifts are reflected in higher consumption of proteins, sugars, fats, and vegetables (Gaiha *et al.* 2013b).

Some of the underlying factors include expansion of the middle class, higher female participation, emergence of nuclear two-income families, a sharp age-divide in food preferences, with younger age-groups more susceptible to new foods advertised in the media, and a rapid growth of super markets and fast-food outlets.[1]

Dietary changes observed since the 1980s (based on Food and Agriculture Organization Statistical Databases [FAOSTAT])[2] are delineated below:

- During the 1980s, consumption of both animal and vegetable products rose sharply; among animal products, the largest proportional

* Reprinted from *Journal of Asian and African Studies*, vol. 48, no. 3, R. Gaiha, R. Jha, and V.S. Kulkarni, 'How Pervasive is Eating Out in India?', pp. 370–86, 2013, with permission from SAGE Publications Ltd.

increase was in the consumption of milk; and among vegetable products, there were large increases in rice, pulses, wheat, spices, and oils.[3]

- During the 1990s, the pattern of food consumption changed significantly; there was a marked increase in the consumption of animal products—especially animal fats—but a relatively modest increase in that of vegetable products; among the latter, there were large increases in the consumption of wheat, starchy roots, vegetable oils, sugar and sweeteners, and fruits, while that of rice, pulses, and other cereals declined; among the starchy roots, potato recorded a sharp increase given its salience in energy-dense food products (for example fries and potato chips); and use of wheat changed too, as there is a move away from the traditional *chapatti* to more commercialized and westernized bread products.[4]

As discussed in Chapter 1, the health implications of the dietary transition are not clear-cut.[5] A more varied and nutritionally balanced diet, and higher levels of food hygiene are associated with better health. But there is a trade-off as more energy-dense foods are linked to a higher incidence of diet-related non-communicable diseases (NCDs)—for example diabetes, coronary heart disease, and certain types of cancer.

From this perspective, we report our findings on eating out based on an analysis of a nationwide household survey, *India Human Development Survey 2005* (IHDS), conducted jointly by University of Maryland and National Council of Applied Economic Research (NCAER).

Eating out contributes to diet diversification. It refers to meals or snacks served in restaurants, roadside eating places, tea and snack shops, and street vendors. As the mix of food served includes fast food (burgers, pizzas, *pakora, samosa*), junk food (chips, chocolate, soft drinks), instant foods (noodles, soup powder), and street foods (*chaat, tikki, golgappa*), they are high in sugar, saturated fat, salt, and calorie content, which are associated with higher risks of obesity, hypertension, and impaired glucose tolerance.[6] A related concern is that some of these foods are prepared, handled, and stored in unhygienic conditions that lead to microbiological contamination (Kaushik *et al.* 2011).

The scheme of the chapter is as follows. It describes the data and discusses our findings on the phenomenon of eating out, based on cross-tabulations. It goes on to describe the methodology for the econometric analysis and gives the empirical results, followed by certain concluding remarks.

DATA

IHDS covers over 41,000 households residing in rural and urban areas, selected from thirty-three states.[7] The sample comprises 384 districts out of a total of 593 identified in the 2001 census. Villages and urban blocks constituted the primary sampling unit from which households were selected.

The rural sample contains about half the households that were interviewed initially by NCAER in 1993–4 in a survey entitled 'Human Development Profile of India' (HDPI), and the other half of the sample households was drawn from both districts surveyed in HDPI, as well as from districts located in the states and union territories not covered in HDPI. The original HDPI was a random sample of 33,230 households located in sixteen major states, 195 districts, and 1,765 villages. In states where the 1993–4 survey was conducted and the contact details were available, 13,593 households were randomly selected for re-interview in 2005. About 82 per cent of the households were contactable for re-interview, resulting in a survey of 11,153 original households as well as 2,440 households, which had separated from the original households, but were still living in the same village.

In each district where re-interviews were conducted, two fresh villages were randomly selected using a probability proportional to size technique. In each village, twenty randomly selected households were chosen. Additionally, 3,993 households were randomly selected from the states where the 1993–4 survey was not conducted, or where contact information was not available.

In order to draw a random sample of urban households, all urban areas in a state were listed in the order of their size, with number of blocks drawn from each urban area allocated based on probability proportional to size. After determining the number of blocks, the enumeration blocks were selected randomly. From these enumeration blocks (of about 150–200 households), a complete household listing was obtained and a sample of fifteen households was selected per block.

Comparison of IHDS data with the National Sample Survey or NSS (2004–5), National Family Health Survey III or NFHS-III (2005–6), and Census (2001) confirms the robustness of IHDS data. For example, IHDS sample distribution on urban residence, caste, and religion is remarkably similar to NSS and NFHS-III, although all three surveys (IHDS, NSS, and NFHS) have higher proportions of households claiming Scheduled Caste (SC) status than enumerated in Census (2001).

SOCIO-ECONOMIC AND SPATIAL CHARACTERISTICS OF HOUSEHOLDS EATING OUT

Our focus is on the socio-economic status of households eating out, and their spatial distribution. The latter disaggregates household locations into rural and urban areas, and urban slums. A further disaggregation separates six metros from the rest. Eating out refers to meals or snacks served in restaurants, roadside eating places, tea and snack shops, and food vendors. A selection of cross-tabulations is given below: relating to location (rural, urban, urban slums, metros), socio-economic characteristics of those eating out, and the amounts spent.

Location

Table 4.1 gives the distribution of households eating out by location. Two different types of locational classification are used: the first distinguishes rural, metros, and non-metro urban areas; and the second distinguishes rural, urban, and urban slums. As illustrated here, eating out is not just a feature of metros or urban areas, but also of urban slums and rural areas. Admittedly, although it is less pervasive in urban slums and rural areas, it is non-negligible. 65.40 per cent of all households that did not eat out lived in rural areas.

The proportion of households eating out is well above one quarter. The highest proportion is found in the six metros, followed by non-metro urban, and rural areas.[8] The differences, however, are small. The differences among the metros are large, with over three-fourths of the households in Bangalore eating out, followed by Chennai, and then Mumbai. At the other extreme are Kolkata (20.13 per cent) and Delhi (about 25 per cent). Another locational classification further corroborates

TABLE 4.1 Distribution of Households Eating Out by Location*

	Whether People Ate Out?		
Location	No (%)	Yes (%)	Total (%)
Rural	74.67 (65.40)	25.33 (56.67)	100 (62.94)
Metro	65.54 (9.08)	34.46 (12.19)	100 (9.95)
Non-Metro Urban	67.67 (25.52)	32.33 (31.14)	100 (27.10)
Total	71.86 (100.00)	28.14 (100.00)	100 (100.00)

Source: Authors' calculations based on IHDS, 2005.
Note: *Computations based on IHDS, 2005. Figures in parentheses indicate percentages of total respondents in different cells.

the pervasiveness of eating out—the proportion of households eating out was highest in urban slums (45.9 per cent), followed by urban areas (35.2 per cent), and then rural areas (27.29 per cent).

In the metros, the proportion of non-poor[9] eating out is more than five times higher than that of the poor (36.73 per cent and 7.38 per cent respectively). So clearly, the relatively affluent display a stronger propensity to eat out. However, while it is not surprising that the proportion of non-poor eating out in non-metros is markedly lower (31.30 per cent), that of the poor is higher (13.84 per cent). As we are unable to probe the quality and price differences, these may be key to the narrower gap between proportions of non-poor and poor eating out in non-metros.

As economic deprivation is highest among the STs, followed by the SCs, and then OBCs, the cross-classification of households affiliated to these groups by whether they ate out is revealing (Gaiha *et al.* 2008). The proportion eating out was highest among the STs, followed by the OBCs, and then 'others' (Table 4.2). So the convenience and cheapness of eating out are presumably inducing relatively deprived households and/or those living in deprived areas to turn to this option in large numbers.

Whether the decision to eat out is linked to the family type—nuclear or joint—is sought to be captured in the cross-tabulation in Table 4.3.[10]

TABLE 4.2 Distribution of Households Eating Out by Caste*

Caste	Whether People Ate Out?		
	No (%)	Yes (%)	Total (%)
Scheduled Castes (SCs)	75.57	24.43	100
	(22.14)	(17.0)	(20.61)
Scheduled Tribes (STs)	71.46	28.54	100
	(7.39)	(7.0)	(7.28)
Other Backward Castes (OBCs)	68.22	31.78	100
	(34.97)	(38.61)	(36.06)
Others	69.26	30.74	100
	(35.50)	(37.39)	(36.05)
Total	70.35	29.65	100
	(100)	(100)	(100)

Source: Authors' calculations based on IHDS, 2005.
Note: *Computed from IHDS, 2005. Figures in parentheses indicate percentages of total respondents in different cells.

TABLE 4.3 Distribution of Households Eating Out by Family Type*

Family Type	Whether People Ate Out?		
	No (%)	Yes (%)	Total (%)
Nuclear	72.16	27.84	100
	(53.03)	(52.43)	(52.86)
Joint	69.88	30.12	100
	(38.17)	(42.16)	(39.29)
Other	80.63	19.37	100
	(8.81)	(5.42)	(7.86)
Total	71.93	28.07	100
	(100)	(100)	(100)

Source: Authors' calculations based on IHDS, 2005.
Note: *Calculations based on IHDS, 2005. Figures in parentheses indicate percentages of total respondents in different cells.

About 28 per cent of nuclear families ate out as compared to a slightly higher share of joint families. The corresponding proportion of the residual group was considerably lower (over 19 per cent). Among those who ate out, more than 50 per cent belonged to nuclear families, and a little under half to joint families. If joint families displayed a stronger propensity to eat out, it could be in part a manifestation of diverse living arrangements (for example, some relatives may simply live under the same roof but may not share meals).

Let us now turn to cross-tabulations of expenditure on eating out and socio-economic status of households. In Table 4.4, a cross-tabulation of eating out (monthly) expenditure by monthly (household) per capita expenditure is given.[11] Note that the poverty cut-off point for the major states lie in the monthly per capita expenditure (MPCE) range—Rs 300–500. So those in the lower range may be described as acutely or extremely poor, while those in the range >Rs 1000 as relatively affluent.

One striking feature is that the proportion of households eating out rises among the three lowest expenditure ranges, and then falls sharply in the highest range (>Rs 1000). Another striking result is that amounts spent vary in a somewhat complex fashion. If we consider those in extreme or moderate poverty (that is, the first two monthly expenditure ranges), small or moderately high fractions of households spending small amounts on eating out fall sharply. In the intermediate

TABLE 4.4 Distribution of Household Expenditure on Eating Out by Monthly Per Capita Expenditure (MPCE) (in Rs)*

Eating Out (Rs)	<300	300–500	500–1000	>1000	Total
None	12.82	28.71	38.40	20.07	100
	(87.52)	(79.19)	(68.20)	(57.44)	(70.35)
1–99	8.57	27.55	44.84	19.03	100
	(10.37)	(13.47)	(14.12)	(9.66)	(12.47)
100–199	2.24	16.87	49.04	31.85	100
	(1.85)	(5.61)	(10.50)	(10.99)	(8.48)
200–499	0.39	6.18	37.71	55.72	100
	(0.25)	(1.59)	(6.25)	(14.89)	(6.57)
>500	0.10	1.69	17.14	81.08	100
	(0.02)	(0.14)	(0.92)	(7.03)	(2.13)
Total	10.30	25.51	39.61	24.58	100
	(100)	(100)	(100)	(100)	(100)

Source: Authors' calculations based on IHDS, 2005.

Note: *Calculations based on IHDS, 2005. Figures in parentheses indicate percentage of total respondents in different cells.

range of monthly expenditure (Rs 500–1000), the proportions spending small to moderate amounts is higher and a non-negligible proportion spend more than moderate amounts on eating out. In the highest expenditure range or among the relatively affluent (with a monthly per capita expenditure >Rs 1000), there is a clear progression of proportions spending larger amounts on eating out except in the highest range of eating out expenditure (>Rs 500). But even in this cell, the share of the relatively affluent is non-negligible (about 7 per cent). So the upshot is that relatively affluent are more likely to eat out, as also to spend larger amounts.

This comes out more sharply in the sub-sample for the metros. Among the relatively affluent; for example, the proportion spending larger amounts on eating out rises from over 6 per cent to about 18 per cent, but falls to about 12 per cent in the highest eating out expenditure range (>Rs 500). In case of metros, while the proportion spending larger amounts on eating out decreases sharply among the poor, there is a progression among the non-poor—except in the highest range of eating out expenditure. In the non-metro sub-sample, however, while the proportion of poor spending larger amounts drops sharply, it also falls among the non-poor, but more slowly.

As monthly per capita expenditure is only a proxy for the standard of living, it is worthwhile to examine linkages between eating out and castes—some of which are highly poverty prone (see Table 4.5). Two remarks are in order; one that proportions of those eating out are not higher in all cases in the metros. While those of the SCs and OBCs are higher in the metros—especially of the latter—that of the STs is much higher in the non-metros. The second remark is that the amounts spent by each of these deprived groups—with varying degrees of deprivation—are higher in the metros. So it follows that even relatively deprived groups are not immune to changing lifestyles and dietary changes.

Table 4.6 throws light on eating out amounts in three different locations: rural, urban, and urban slums. The contrast in some respects is striking. The proportions of households spending larger amounts decreases in rural areas, but not so sharply; in the urban areas. By contrast, the proportion of households spending larger amounts rises, but slowly, until the highest eating out expenditure range. In fact, about 16 per cent of the households spend moderately high or high amounts on eating out. But the urban slums are not far behind.

TABLE 4.5 Distribution of Household Expenditure on Eating Out by Caste in Metros*

Eating Out (Rs)	SC	ST	OBC	Others	Total
None	26.59	1.64	25.14	46.63	100
	(73.21)	(82.09)	(60.79)	(66.29)	(66.29)
1–99	25.95	0.28	32.10	41.67	100
	(7.41)	(1.46)	(8.05)	(6.14)	(6.91)
100–199	24.62	0.96	39.62	34.80	100
	(10.80)	(7.66)	(15.27)	(7.88)	(10.62)
200–499	16.20	0.47	31.20	52.13	100
	(7.02)	(3.67)	(11.88)	(11.67)	(10.50)
>500	7.12	1.29	20.80	70.80	100
	(1.56)	(5.13)	(4.0)	(8.01)	(5.68)
Total	24.21	1.33	27.56	46.89	100
	(100)	(100)	(100)	(100)	(100)

Source: Authors' calculations based on IHDS, 2005.
Note: *Calculations based on IHDS, 2005. Figures in parentheses indicate percentages of total respondents in different cells.

TABLE 4.6 Distribution of Household Expenditure on Eating Out by Location*

Eating Out (Rs)	Rural	Urban	Urban Slums	Total
None	74.82	23.88	1.29	100
	(72.71)	(64.80)	(54.10)	(70.35)
1–99	77.45	20.06	2.50	100
	(13.34)	(9.65)	(18.50)	(12.47)
100–199	67.45	29.68	2.86	100
	(7.90)	(9.71)	(14.44)	(8.48)
200–499	54.54	42.45	3.01	100
	(4.95)	(10.75)	(11.76)	(6.57)
>500	37.20	61.86	0.95	100
	(1.10)	(5.09)	(1.20)	(2.13)
Total	72.39	25.93	1.68	100
	(100)	(100)	(100)	(100)

Source: Authors' calculations based on IHDS, 2005.
Note: *Calculations based on IHDS, 2005. Figures in parentheses indicate percentage of total respondents in that category.

About 33 per cent of the households spent small or slightly larger amounts, but about 14 per cent also spent moderately high or high amounts. As noted already, even deprived locations are not immune to lifestyle changes and convenience of eating out.

We constructed cross-classifications of household expenditure on eating out by type of family in the aggregate sample, metros, and rural areas respectively (Table 4.7). Among those who eat out in nuclear families, there is a steady decrease in the share of households as expenditure on eating out rises. In fact, a large majority of these (76 per cent) spent small amounts (<Rs 200) while the remaining spent more (>Rs 200). The pattern is similar among joint families. About 71 per cent spent small amounts (<Rs 200), and the remaining moderate amounts (>Rs 200).

If these results are compared with those for the metros, the patterns are different. It is not just that more nuclear families eat out, they also tend to spend larger amounts in the metros (relative to the aggregate sample). About 50 per cent of these spent small amounts (<Rs 200), while about 17 per cent spent large amounts (>Rs 500). Among the

TABLE 4.7 Distribution of Expenditure on Eating Out by Family Type (Aggregate)*

Eating Out (Rs)	Nuclear	Joint	Other	Total
None	53.03	38.17	8.81	100
	(72.16)	(69.88)	(80.63)	(71.93)
1–99	55.79	38.15	6.07	100
	(13.67)	(12.58)	(10.01)	(12.95)
100–199	50.59	44.04	5.36	100
	(7.42)	(8.69)	(5.29)	(7.75)
200–499	48.08	47.57	4.35	100
	(5.18)	(6.90)	(3.16)	(5.70)
>500	49.70	46.01	4.29	100
	(1.57)	(1.95)	(0.91)	(1.67)
Total	52.86	39.29	7.86	100
	(100)	(100)	(100)	(100)

Source: Authors' calculations based on IHDS, 2005.

Note: *Calculations based on IHDS, 2005. Figures in parentheses indicate percentages of total respondents in different cells.

joint families, a considerably higher proportion ate out. However, about half spent small amounts (<Rs 200) while over 16 per cent spent large amounts (>Rs 500). So more joint families in the metros ate out and spent larger amounts too, as compared with the aggregate sample. In the rural areas, about the same proportion of nuclear and joint families (about 25 per cent) ate out and large majorities (84 per cent and 78 per cent, respectively) spent small amounts, while a larger segment of the latter spent amounts exceeding Rs 200.

In sum, eating out is a pervasive phenomenon—especially in the urban areas and, more specifically, in the metros. While relatively affluent are more prone to eating out and spend larger amounts, some of the deprived segments, using not just income/expenditure criteria, but also caste and location, do not seem to lag far behind. Eating out is not merely an urban phenomenon, as large segments in rural areas eat out too.

METHODOLOGY

While these cross-tabulations yielded some insights into the pervasiveness of the eating out phenomenon, the 'marginal' contributions of household traits—including their poverty status, demographic composition, whether a nuclear or a joint family—and locational effects could not be assessed. To do so, we have experimented with the Heckman selection model. This comprises of two stages: (i) the decision to eat out is analysed, and (ii) this is followed by how amounts spent on eating out vary with household and other characteristics.

As detailed expositions of the Heckman model are available in various text books, we draw upon Wooldridge (2006). The approach to incidental truncation is to add an explicit selection equation to the population model of interest:

$$y = \mathbf{x}\boldsymbol{\beta} + u, E(u|x) = 0 \tag{1}$$

$$s = 1[\mathbf{z}\boldsymbol{\gamma} + v \geq 0] \tag{2}$$

where s = 1 if we observe y, and 0 otherwise. As the elements of x and z are always observed, we write $\boldsymbol{x\beta} = \beta_0 + \beta_1 x_1 + \cdots \beta_k x_k$ and $\boldsymbol{z\gamma} = \gamma_0 + \gamma_1 z_1 + \cdots \gamma_m z_m$. The equation of primary interest is (1), and $\boldsymbol{\beta}$

could be estimated by ordinary least squares (OLS) given a random sample. The selection equation, (2), depends on observed variables, z_h, and an unobserved error, v. Exogeneity of **z** implies E(u | **x**,**z**) = 0. In fact, for the model that we propose to estimate, **x** must be a subset of **z**.

The error term ν in the sample selection equation is assumed to be independent of **z** (and therefore **x**). It is also assumed that v has a standard normal distribution. Any correlation between u and ν causes a sample selection problem.

As u and ν are related, and ν has a standard normal distribution, it is easy to show that E (ν | **z**, s) is simply the inverse Mills ratio, $\boldsymbol{\lambda}(\mathbf{z}\boldsymbol{\gamma})$, when s = 1. (Wooldridge 2006). This leads to the important equation,

$$E\left(y\middle|\mathbf{z},s\right) = \mathbf{x}\boldsymbol{\beta} + \rho E\left(v\middle|\mathbf{z},s\right) \quad (3)$$

Equation (3) shows that expected value of y, given **z**, and observability of y is equal to $\mathbf{x}\boldsymbol{\beta}$, plus an additional term that depends on the inverse Mills ratio evaluated at $\mathbf{z}\boldsymbol{\gamma}$. This equation shows that we can estimate $\boldsymbol{\beta}$ by using only the selected sample, provided we include $\boldsymbol{\gamma}(\mathbf{z}\boldsymbol{\gamma})$ as an additional regressor.

If $\rho = 0$, $\boldsymbol{\lambda}(\mathbf{zy})$ does not appear, OLS of y on **x** using the selected sample consistently estimates $\boldsymbol{\beta}$ Otherwise, effectively the variable, $\boldsymbol{\lambda}(\mathbf{zy})$, correlated with **x**, is omitted. $\rho = 0$ when u and ν are uncorrelated.

Since λ is unknown, we cannot evaluate $\boldsymbol{\lambda}(\mathbf{z}_i\boldsymbol{\gamma})$ for each *i*. However, given the assumptions, and with *s* also given, *z* follows a probit model

$$P\left(s=1\middle|\mathbf{z}\right) = \boldsymbol{\Phi}\left(\mathbf{z}\boldsymbol{\gamma}\right) \quad (4)$$

So $\boldsymbol{\gamma}$ is estimated by probit of s_i on $\mathbf{z}_i$, using the entire sample. In a second step, $\boldsymbol{\beta}$ is estimated from a regression of y_i on $\mathbf{x}_i$, $\hat{\boldsymbol{\lambda}}_i$, using the selected sample for which $s_i = 1$. The $\hat{\beta}_j$ are consistent and approximately normally distributed. The *t* statistic on $\hat{\lambda}_i$ tests $H_0 = 0$. Under H_0 there is no selection bias.

An alternative to this two-step estimation is full maximum likelihood estimation. This requires obtaining the joint distribution of y and s. Usually, the two-step procedure is applied first to test for selection bias. After the selection bias is confirmed, the regression and selection equation are estimated jointly by MLE (Wooldridge 2006).[12]

EMPIRICAL RESULTS

As the two-step procedure rejects the null, $H_0=0$ shown in Table 4.8, our comments are confined to the MLE results in Table 4.9. This is standard procedure.[13]

TABLE 4.8 Heckman Selection Model—Two-Step Estimates

Heckman selection model—two-step estimates (regression model with sample selection)	Number of obs = 41349 Censored obs = 29697 Uncensored obs = 11652 Wald chi2(20) = 1977.64 Prob>chi2 = 0.0000			
	Coef.	Std. Err.	z	P>z
Eating out—Rupees				
Metro	97.410	9.153	10.640***	0.000
Urban	17.136	6.650	2.580***	0.010
SC/ST	−38.290	6.759	−5.670***	0.000
OBC	−57.634	6.224	−9.260***	0.000
Expenditure Poverty Ratio	17.299	1.543	11.210***	0.000
No. of adult males in paid work age group 18–24	−6.422	6.544	−0.980	0.326
No. of adult males in paid work age group 25–45	6.750	5.047	1.340	0.181
No. of adult males in paid work age group >45	11.140	6.467	1.720*	0.085
share of salary in total income	−0.474	0.345	−1.370	0.170
share of business income in total income	0.467	0.122	3.820***	0.000
Constant	429.472	36.463	11.780	0.000
Eating out (0/1)				
Metro	0.208	0.023	9.010***	0.000
Urban	0.186	0.016	11.640***	0.000
Nuclear family	0.274	0.028	9.710***	0.000
Joint family	0.368	0.029	12.720***	0.000
SC/ST	−0.041	0.018	−2.320**	0.021
OBC	0.112	0.016	7.050***	0.000
Expenditure Poverty Ratio	0.093	0.003	30.490***	0.000

(continued)

TABLE 4.8 Continued

Heckman selection model—two-step estimates (regression model with sample selection)	Number of obs = 41349 Censored obs = 29697 Uncensored obs = 11652 Wald chi2(20) = 1977.64 Prob>chi2 = 0.0000			
	Coef.	Std. Err.	z	P>z
No. of adult males in paid work age group 18–24	0.089	0.017	5.150***	0.000
No. of adult males in paid work age group 25–45	0.077	0.013	6.060***	0.000
No. of adult males in paid work age group >45	−0.008	0.018	−0.450	0.651
No. of adult females in paid work age group 18–24	0.160	0.028	5.670***	0.000
No. of adult females in paid work age group 25–45	0.135	0.017	8.090***	0.000
No. of adult females in paid work age group >45	−0.017	0.028	−0.600	0.550
Share of salary in total income	0.125	0.017	7.580***	0.000
Share of business income in total income	0.001	0.001	2.290*	0.022
Constant	−1.304	0.031	−41.930	0.000
lambda	−256.968	24.871	−10.330***	0.000
rho	−0.798			
sigma	321.837			
lambda	−256.968	24.871		

Source: Authors' calculations based on IHDS, 2005.
Note: *** denote significance at the 1 per cent level, ** at the 5 per cent level, and * at the 10 per cent level.

Let us first consider the probit results. The main findings are: both metro and non-metro urban locations induce eating out, relative to the rural. As lifestyle changes in these locations have been more dramatic and convenience of eating out is greater, these are plausible results. Both nuclear and joint families display higher propensities to eat out relative to others. Between the two, joint families are more likely to eat out. While the coefficient of SCs/STs is negative, it is

TABLE 4.9 Heckman Selection Model—MLE Results

Heckman selection model (regression model with sample selection) Log pseudo likelihood = -4.74e+08	Number of obs = 41349 Censored obs = 29697 Uncensored obs = 11652 Wald chi2(10) = 548.52 Prob>chi2 = 0.0000			
	Coef.	Robust Std. Err	Z	P>|z|
Eating out—Rupees				
Metro	104.224	11.270	9.250***	0.000
Urban	47.152	5.800	8.130***	0.000
SC/ST	−45.254	5.103	−8.870***	0.000
OBC	−37.580	8.517	−4.410***	0.000
Expenditure Poverty Ratio	26.574	2.653	10.020***	0.000
No. of adult males in paid work age group 18–24	5.280	5.652	0.930	0.350
No. of adult males in paid work age group 25–45	19.953	5.857	3.410***	0.000
No. of adult males in paid work age group >45	20.976	13.918	1.510^{W}	0.130
share of salary in total income	−0.205	0.105	−1.960**	0.050
share of business income in total income	0.536	0.342	1.570^{W}	0.120
Constant	121.251	14.764	8.210***	0.000
Eating out (0/1)				
Metro	0.150	0.039	3.840	0.000
Urban	0.201	0.020	9.870***	0.000
Nuclear family	0.285	0.041	7.000***	0.000
Joint family	0.401	0.042	9.460***	0.000
SC/ST	−0.037	0.025	−1.500^{W}	0.130
OBC	0.097	0.023	4.180***	0.000
Expenditure Poverty Ratio	0.119	0.007	16.820***	0.000
No. of adult males in paid work age group 18–24	0.097	0.024	4.040***	0.000
No. of adult males in paid work age group 25–45	0.099	0.019	5.110***	0.000

(continued)

TABLE 4.9 Continued

Heckman selection model (regression model with sample selection) Log pseudo likelihood = -4.74e+08	Number of obs = 41349 Censored obs = 29697 Uncensored obs = 11652 Wald chi2(10) = 548.52 Prob>chi2 = 0.0000			
	Coef.	Robust Std. Err	Z	P>|z|
No. of adult males in paid work age group >45	0.025	0.030	0.850	0.400
No. of adult females in paid work age group 18–24	0.172	0.045	3.850***	0.000
No. of adult females in paid work age group 25–45	0.112	0.025	4.570***	0.000
No. of adult females in paid work age group >45	−0.018	0.040	−0.440	0.660
Share of salary in total income	0.166	0.031	5.400***	0.000
Share of business income in total income	0.001	0.001	1.300	0.190
Constant	−1.376	0.047	−29.360	0.000
/athrho	−0.224	0.041	−5.450	0.000
/lnsigma	5.392	0.082	65.950	0.000
rho	−0.220	0.039		
sigma	219.731	17.966		
lambda	−48.448	6.924***		

Source: Authors' calculations based on IHDS, 2005.
Note: Wald test of indep. eqns. (rho = 0): chi2 (1) = 29.75. Prob > chi2 = 0.0000.
*** Denote significance at the 1 per cent level, ** at the 5 per cent level, and * at the 10 per cent level.

weakly significant, implying a lower propensity to eat out, relative to the omitted group of 'others'. That of OBCs is positive and significant, suggesting that they are more likely to eat out. The higher the number of adult males in paid work in the two age groups, 18 to 24 years, and 25 to 45 years, the greater is the likelihood of such households eating out. The same applies to the number of adult females in paid employment in these age groups. Control for the effects of these and other right side variables, the higher the ratio of per capita expenditure to the poverty cut-off expenditure, the higher is the probability of such households eating out. This confirms the important role of growing affluence in dietary changes. We have further examined whether the sources of income matter too. The higher the share of salary in household income, the greater is the likelihood of eating out. While the effect of higher share of business income is positive too, it is weakly significant.

Turning to the factors underlying the eating out expenditure, our main results are the following: location matters a great deal. Households located in both metros and non-metro urban locations are likely to spend larger amounts on eating out, relative to rural areas.

Between the metros and non-metros, households in the former are likely to spend much larger amounts. Both SCs/STs and OBCs are likely to spend lower amounts relative to 'others'. The higher the number of adult males in paid employment in the age group 25 to 45, the greater is the amount spent. A similar result is obtained for the number of adults in paid employment in the older age group, >45 years, but the coefficient is only weakly significant. The effect of higher per capita expenditure relative to the poverty line is large and significant, confirming that the more affluent are not just likely to eat out more often but also likely to spend larger amounts. Somewhat surprisingly, the higher the share of salary in household income, the lower is the amount spent. By contrast, the higher the share of business income, the larger is the amount spent.

In sum, most of the results are plausible. Specifically, location of households, their demographic and caste characteristics, and above all, their relative affluence influence both the decision to eat out, and, conditional on it, the amount spent.

★★★

The main findings are summarized from a broad policy perspective. Attention was drawn to growing affluence, urbanization, and dietary changes that are occurring at a rapid pace in developing countries. Of particular significance in the Indian context is the expansion of the middle class, higher female participation, emergence of nuclear two-income families, a sharp age-divide in food preferences with younger age groups more susceptible to new foods advertized in the media, and a rapid growth of super markets and fast food outlets.

There have been concomitant changes in dietary patterns. Consumption of animal products—especially fats—has increased, but that of vegetable products only moderately. Among the latter, consumption of wheat, starchy roots, vegetable oils, sweets and sweeteners, and fruits has increased while that of cereals and pulses has declined.[14] Also, the forms in which some of these products are consumed has changed—chapatti, for example, is increasingly replaced by commercialized and westernized bread products.

Viewed from this perspective, our analysis broadly confirms the important role of urbanization, demographic changes, expansion of middle class, and its growing affluence in eating out, or more generally, consumption of snacks, beverages, and pre-cooked meals. To the extent that even more deprived sections are not immune to these evolving dietary patterns, and given their limited access to medical care and dietary awareness, the health outcomes may well be a lot grimmer than often acknowledged.

NOTES

1. For an admirably lucid exposition of growth of supermarkets and fast food outlets, and shifts in dietary patterns, see Timmer (2009). On the latter, also see Shetty *et al.* (2002) and Reddy *et al.* (2005).
2. For details, see Pingali (2007), and Pingali and Khwaja (2004). For a more recent analysis, based on several rounds of the NSS household surveys, pointing to a downward shift of the calorie Engle consumption curve, see Deaton and Dréze (2009). Their conjecture that a major explanatory factor is improvement in social epidemiology of disease, easier access to drinking water, and transportation facilities is subject to careful scrutiny. A related study focusing on nutrition-poverty link is Mahal and Karan (2008). For an alternative view emphasizing nutrition-poverty traps, see Jha *et al.* (2009a).
3. Note that in our classification, vegetables are defined narrowly; for example, cereals, pulses, edible oils are excluded.
4. FAO's estimate of food consumption are obtained from its availability, and thus not directly comparable with actual food consumption data collected by the NSS and IHDS, 2005.
5. For a sample of contributions to diet-related NCDs, see Mahal *et al.* (2009), Mahal and Karan (2008), and Popkin *et al.* (2001).

6. Note that these are distinct categories, but with some overlap. Hence, fast food is subsumed to include others for expositional convenience.
7. This is a summary of the material provided by Sonal Desai.
8. The six metros are Bangalore, Kolkata, Chennai, Delhi, Mumbai, and Hyderabad.
9. The poverty line used is the official poverty line in terms of monthly per capita expenditure. For details, see Himanshu (2007).
10. A nuclear family is one that includes a married couple, with or without both spouses living together, and their children, if any. A joint family includes other relatives. Other cases (for example, a widow/widower, or a separated spouse living alone) are combined in the residual group.
11. Since household food consumption is influenced more by total amount spent eating out as opposed to per capita amounts, we preferred the former.
12. Adkins and Hill (2008) also recommend the MLE procedure. They observe, 'In most instances, it is preferable to estimate the full model, both the selection equation and the equation of interest, jointly by maximum likelihood' (p. 399).
13. As $\hat{\lambda}_i$ is significantly different from 0, there is selection bias. So the two-step Heckman model estimation is followed by maximum likelihood estimation.
14. Sugar consumed through sweets and beverages is not included in the consumption of sugar. Hence moderate reduction in sugar consumption during 1993–2004 is suspect.

5 Calorie Thresholds and Undernutrition in India, 1993–2004*

Nidhi Kaicker and Raghav Gaiha

In India, despite rising incomes, there has been a sustained decline in per capita calorie intake.[1] If the proportions of undernourished are measured using fixed calorie norms, there is an increase in the prevalence of undernutrition (synonymous with calorie-deprivation). Even if the calorie norms are taken to be lower, as illustrated later, a grim picture emerges. A recent contribution (Jensen and Miller 2011) is deeply sceptical of such norms for familiar reasons (detailed later in this chapter, in Results) and proposes an alternative measure that relies on consumption behaviour, as opposed to calorie norms. The basic argument is that individuals tend to switch away from the cheapest source of calories (staple food sources), after surpassing subsistence, towards more expensive sources of calories. If this switch occurs at a certain share of calories from staples, all those above the threshold are counted as undernourished. An application to China reveals a huge difference between proportions of undernourished, measured using fixed calorie norms and the behavioural approach just delineated.

This motivated our analysis with the National Sample Survey (NSS) data for 1993 and 2004. As the continuing food price spiral has

* Reprinted from *Journal of Policy Modeling*, vol. 35, no. 2, N. Kaicker and R. Gaiha, 'Calorie Thresholds and Undernutrition in India, 1993–2004', pp. 271–88, March–April 2013, with permission from Elsevier Limited.

reignited fears of another crisis with dire consequences for the poor, it is vital for policy purposes to get the measurement of undernutrition right. This concern is reinforced by a national debate on universalizing the food subsidy through the public distribution system (PDS). While the case for a universal food subsidy is weak and controversial given huge losses from the PDS, food security nevertheless remains an overriding policy concern (discussed in Chapter 9). We first review the Jensen and Miller study (2011) in this chapter, and then discuss some analytical and interpretational issues. Our methodology is detailed, followed by the results and concluding observations.

CALORIE THRESHOLDS

Jensen and Miller (2011) invoke several familiar arguments against using fixed calorie norms.[2] These include: (i) lack of a consensus on what the correct minimum calorie threshold is, how it should be computed, or even whether such a threshold exists (Dasgupta 1995; Srinivasan, 1993; Svedberg 2000); (ii) as calorie norms vary by age, sex, health status, activity patterns, and basal metabolic rate—some of which are unobservable or too difficult to measure—use of standardized norms to measure undernutrition is problematic; (iii) not all nutrients consumed are absorbed before leaving the body. One difficulty in absorption is high incidence of diseases such as diarrhoea. But even in the absence of such diseases, absorption rates vary between individuals. This introduces a 'noise' in the measurement of undernutrition, as individuals may appear to consume far more than their 'true needs', absorbing only a fraction of that amount; and (iv) there is a large literature confirming that, as household incomes rise, households tend to substitute towards foods with non-nutritional attributes (for example, taste for variety).[3] Such behaviour reflects a weaker preference for calories than for taste.

Jensen and Miller (2011) accordingly propose and implement an alternative measure based on calorie share of staples threshold. The calorie share of staples is divided by total calories consumed. Over a range, the consumer prefers staples and after a certain wealth she/he switches to other more expensive sources of calories. This switch point of calorie share from staples is the threshold.[4] This is rationalized on the following grounds: (i) an individual before attaining this threshold experiences physical sensations of hunger: headaches, pain, dizziness, and failure to concentrate; (ii) as the marginal utility of additional calories is high, a utility maximizing consumer concentrates on consuming calories from the cheapest sources (rice, wheat, or cassava). However, after crossing the calorie threshold at higher wealth, the consumer begins to substitute towards more expensive sources of calories (meat, fruits, and vegetables) and a more varied diet. Thus, at the threshold, the marginal utility of calories is low and subsistence is surpassed.

Apart from overcoming the difficulties arising from individual-specific and unobservable subsistence thresholds, it is claimed that the proposed measure has the merit of being consistent with revealed consumer preferences, and greater intuitive public policy appeal. The latter lies in a shift from calories to utility.

Jensen and Miller (2011) point out that this threshold matches that computed from the minimum cost diet problem, subject, of course, to the caveat that such diets are seldom consumed by the impoverished (Deaton 1995). Besides, they report that their threshold is very stable with respect to factors such as age, height, weight, and activity level. So, based on their analysis with Chinese data, the threshold follows a tight range that helps 'identify hunger across all individuals, regardless of their attributes' (Deaton 1995: 4).

There are a few limitations of this measure, however. These include (i) omission of other nutrients; (ii) failure to account for long-term adjustment of the human body to nutritional deprivation; and (iii) lack of sensitivity to the depth of deprivation.

As argued and illustrated below, there appear to be more serious flaws in this measure.

In trying to replicate and refine the Jensen and Miller (2011) results, we first employ Lowess regressions of calorie share of cereals (wheat, rice, and inferior cereals that account for a large share of total calories) on a measure of wealth (monthly per capita expenditure or MPCE), followed by an expanded specification in which, along with food prices, demographic and caste variables are used as explanatory variables.[5] Changes in the calorie share thresholds and corresponding expenditures/incomes are striking. More striking are the changes in the proportions of undernourished.

While the Lowess results, as discussed later, largely corroborate the Jensen and Miller hypothesis, they raise a few analytical concerns discussed below:

1. Underlying the empirical analysis is a utility maximizing model, net of a penalty function, with a budget constraint.[6] The reduced form of calorie share as a function of wealth (approximated by income), estimated using Lowess, suggests that over a range of wealth, the consumer prefers staples to any other food commodity until the threshold level is reached. Arguably, this is also consistent with lexicographic ordering of consumer preferences for staples. In that case, following Cantor's theorem, it cannot be represented by a real valued utility function.
2. In an important paper, Timmer (1981) estimated curvature in the Slutsky matrix, based on the 1976 Socio-Economic Survey—Susenas V—for Indonesia. Or, more specifically, the question addressed is whether the Slutsky substitution elasticities vary by income class? Whether the poor exhibit higher or lower substitution elasticities than others in a context of spiralling food prices—ignored in the Jensen and Miller analysis (2011)—is of considerable significance in understanding the extent and severity of undernutrition.
3. In another important contribution, Behrman and Deolalikar (1989) examine the conjecture that food variety *per se* is valued so that people purchase food variety as their incomes rise, while calorie intakes change slightly. They focus on two characteristics of consumer preferences over different foods: the degree of curvature and centrality (relative to the axes) of the location of food indifference curves. If low cost calories dominate food choices at very low incomes, the food indifference curves are likely to be relatively flat (so price induced substitution is high) and located closer to the axis for the cheapest source of calories. As incomes and food budgets increase, food indifference curves may be more sharply curved and centred far away from the cheapest source of calories' axis. The analysis is based on the ICP data on thirty-four countries for 1975, and on sixty countries for 1980. Two results are particularly relevant here: (i) for the poorest sub-sample of countries, the food indifference curves are considerably flatter than the Cobb-Douglas case. However, for the next sub-sample, there is greater curvature of

the food indifference curves. Hence, as food budgets increase, demand for food variety rises, with the food indifference curves changing from flat to being L-shaped; (ii) the implied (relative prices-constant) ratios of breads/cereals to most other foods consumed either falls or remains unchanged between the poorest sub-sample and the next. Since breads/cereals are the cheapest source of calories, it follows that as food expenditures and incomes increase from very low levels, there is evidence of a locational shift of the food indifference curves away from the axis of the cheapest source of calories and towards other foods given constant relative prices. Two points emerge from this analysis: one is a strong relative price effect among the poor, and the other is the strong income effect. Neglect of the former in the Jensen and Miller analysis (2011) is thus limiting.

4. Characterization of the undernourished as those with calorie share of staples above the threshold is somewhat arbitrary and ambiguous. Consider Figure 5.1, which resembles the Lowess curves reported in Jensen and Miller (2011). As also illustrated with India's NSS data, there are four sections on the basis of calorie and wealth thresholds. Jensen and Miller (2011) take the fraction of the population above the calorie threshold as the undernourished. The level

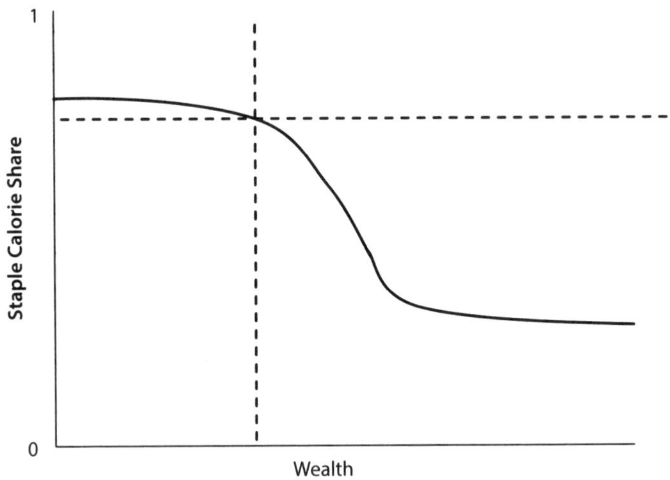

FIGURE 5.1 Staple Calorie Share and Wealth
Source: Authors' calculations based on NSS (50th and 61st rounds).

of wealth/income corresponding to the calorie threshold ceases to have any significance as all those on either side of the wealth cut-off, but above the calorie threshold, are added up. What is also worrying is exclusion of those below the calorie threshold and to the left of the wealth cut-off.

METHODOLOGY

Here an attempt is made to analyse calorie thresholds with India's NSS household data for 1993 and 2004. As the sample design is identical between these two rounds of the NSS, the results are comparable. The analysis is carried out separately for the rural and urban samples, as consumption patterns differ considerably (Gaiha *et al.* 2012b, 2013b). The calorie conversion was done using recent nutrient-food ratios (Gopalan *et al.* 1971; ICMR 1990). The food commodity classification used is sufficiently disaggregated for analysing switches from largely cereal to more diversified diets.[7] Appropriately weighted food prices at the PSU level were constructed by us.

Following Jensen and Miller (2011), we first experiment with Lowess in which the dependent variable is the share of calories from cereals (cheapest and largest source of calories in India) and the right side variable, wealth of a household per capita, is approximated by monthly per capita expenditure (at 2004 prices). A logarithmic transformation of this variable is used.[8]

The Lowess focuses on the relationship between calorie share of cereals and MPCE. Following our distillation of two important contributions establishing the important role of food prices in inducing substitutions between different sources of calories, we explore with the NSS data how sensitive calorie shares are to food prices, and whether a calorie threshold exists; and in case it does, whether estimates of undernourished change substantially.[9] This analysis is carried out separately for the four NSS samples: rural 1993, rural 2004, urban 1993, and urban 2004.

We use the following specification for our analysis:

$$C_i = \alpha + \beta_1 (\ln Y_i) + \beta_2 (\ln Y_i)^2 + (\ln \boldsymbol{P})\gamma + \delta_1 (HH)$$
$$+ \delta_2 (A) + \boldsymbol{S}\rho + \boldsymbol{C}\varphi + \varepsilon_i$$

where the dependent variable is the proportion of calories obtained from cereals by the ith household, Y_i denotes per capita monthly expenditure, $\boldsymbol{P}$ denotes a vector of food prices, HH denotes household size, A is proportion of adult males in the household, $\boldsymbol{S}$ is a vector of state dummy variables (with Jammu and Kashmir as the omitted state), $\boldsymbol{C}$ is a vector of caste dummy variables (with SCs as the omitted group), and ε_i is the iid (independent and identically distributed variables) error term.

In order to allow for differences in calorie share responses to expenditure and food prices, among other explanatory variables, we have split each sample into two sub-samples comprising the poor and the affluent. These categories are defined in terms of the poverty cut-off points.[10]

RESULTS

Lowess Results

Let us first consider the results for rural India in 1993 and 2004. Figures 5.2 and 5.3 illustrate the Lowess results for rural India for 1993 and 2004. In 1993, the calorie share threshold occurs at 0.80 and the corresponding MPCE is Rs 200.30. Counting those above the threshold (below and above the expenditure threshold), the proportion of undernourished works out to about 27 per cent of the rural population, which is lower than the proportion under the calorie cut-off of 1800 per capita per day. As argued earlier, this estimate of the undernourished lumps together those with incomes below and well above the income threshold. The exclusion of those below the calorie and income thresholds (about 1.2 per cent) seems contentious, if not somewhat arbitrary.

In striking contrast to our analysis with fixed calorie norms, which show a sharp rise in the proportion of undernourished in rural India during 1993–2004, the Lowess results show a substantial reduction, from 27 per cent to 16 per cent. While the calorie threshold is the same (0.80) and the corresponding income is Rs 244.70, much of the reduction is due to a sharp drop in the proportion of those above the threshold and the corresponding expenditure/income. Further, there is also an increase in the proportion of those below the calorie and expenditure thresholds.

Let us now turn to the results for urban India. Figures 5.4 and 5.5 illustrate the Lowess results for urban India for 1993 and 2004.

The calorie threshold in urban India in 1993 is lower than that in rural India, but the expenditure corresponding to the former is slightly higher. However, the proportion of undernourished is a little over half of that for rural India. The majority of the former are those with calorie shares higher than the threshold and expenditures higher than the expenditure threshold. There is a reduction in the proportion of undernourished (from 15 per cent to 9 per cent) due to a sharp reduction in the proportion of those above the calorie threshold and

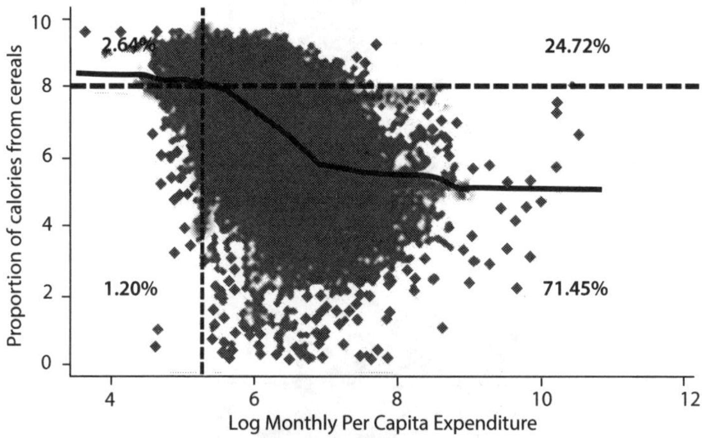

FIGURE 5.2 Distribution of Calories from Cereals for Rural India (1993)
Source: Authors' calculations based on NSS (50th and 61st rounds).

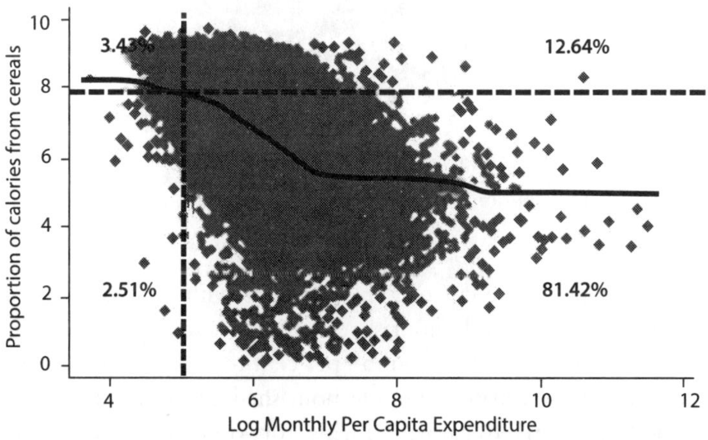

FIGURE 5.3 Distribution of Calories from Cereals for Rural India (2004)
Source: Authors' calculations based on NSS (50th and 61st rounds).

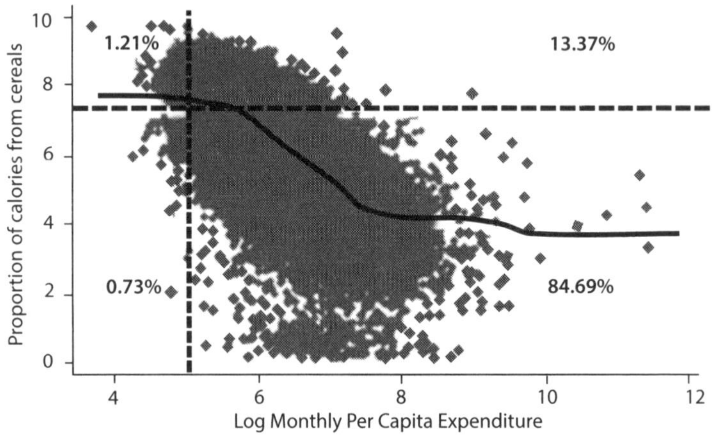

FIGURE 5.4 Distribution of Calories from Cereals for Urban India (1993)
Source: Authors' calculations based on NSS (50th and 61st rounds).

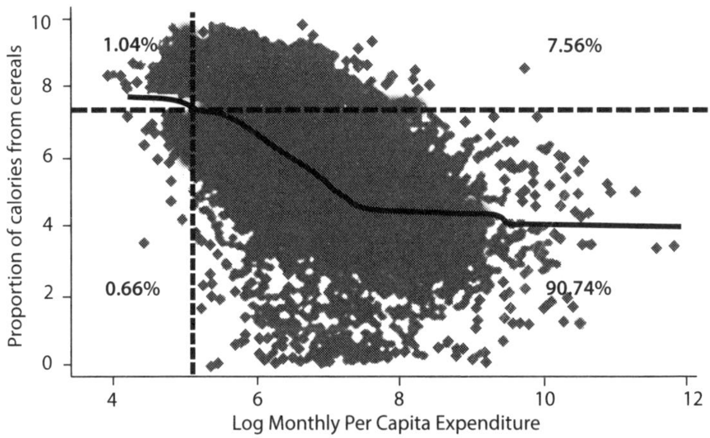

FIGURE 5.5 Distribution of Calories from Cereals for Urban India (2004)

above the expenditure cut-off. This contrasts with the sharp increase in the proportion of undernourished with the calorie cut-off of 2,100 (the proportion rises from about 58 per cent to about 64 per cent).

In sum, the estimates of undernourished are lower than those obtained using fixed calorie norms for rural and urban India. Besides, while Lowess results point to a reduction in the proportion of undernourished over the period 1993–2004—especially in rural India—a sharp rise is observed using fixed calorie cut-off points. Finally, not just lumping together of undernourished below and above the expenditure threshold, but also failure to classify those below both the expenditure and calorie share thresholds weaken the intuitive appeal of the measure of undernutrition proposed by Jensen and Miller (2011).

Calorie Share, Expenditure, and Prices

The robust regression results are discussed below.

RURAL INDIA

Let us first consider the results with the rural India sample for 1993, given in Table 5.1. Among the poor, the calorie share varies with expenditure, and inversely with its square.[11] Demographic variables also influence the calorie share—it rises with household size and proportion of adults. The Scheduled Tribes (STs) and 'others' have lower calorie shares than the Scheduled Castes (SCs). Controlling for these effects, food prices have significant effects on the calorie share: the higher the price of vegetables and meat/poultry/fish, the higher is the share of calories, while the lower the price of pulses/nuts/others and sugar, the higher is this share. Somewhat surprisingly, the price of cereals has a positive impact on this share. These price effects point to substitutes (vegetables, meat/poultry/fish), and complements (pulses/nuts/others, and sugar) in the diets of the acutely poor.

Among the affluent, and in striking contrast to the poor, expenditure has a significant negative effect while its square has a positive effect. Both demographic variables (household size and proportion of adults) have significant positive effects. The STs have a higher calorie share while 'others' have a lower share relative to the SCs. Both prices of Vanaspati oil and pulses/nuts and others have significant negative coefficients, implying that they are complements. Prices of eggs, fruits, and vegetables, by contrast, are positive, implying that they are substitutes. The price of cereals has a positive impact on this share. So, among the affluent too, food prices influence calories from cereals.

Let us now turn to the results from the rural sample for 2004 (Table 5.1). There are some changes—especially in the food price effects.

TABLE 5.1 Regression Results: Rural India (1993 and 2004)

	Poor			Non-Poor			Poor			Non-Poor		
No. of observations	8721			29206			8658			45384		
Prob.>F	0.0000			0.0000			0.0000			0.0000		
	1993						2004					
Log MPCE	0.106	(1.65)	*	−0.480	(−28.55)	***	0.332	(6.07)	***	−0.419	(−41.98)	***
$(\text{Log MPCE})^2$	−0.019	(−3.22)	***	0.027	(21.59)	***	−0.039	(−7.66)	***	0.023	(31.5)	***
Log—Price of Milk & Milk Products	−0.001	(−0.4)	–	−0.001	(−1.02)	–	−0.003	(−2.51)	**	0.006	(8.15)	***
Log—Price of Vanaspati Oil	−0.013	(−1.47)	–	−0.013	(−2.14)	**	0.034	(4.16)	***	0.022	(5.93)	***
Log—Price of Sugar	−0.011	(−1.77)	*	−0.003	(−0.67)	–	−0.006	(−0.97)	–	−0.027	(−8.49)	***
Log—Price of Eggs	−0.001	(−0.28)	–	0.004	(3.27)	***	0.008	(2.71)	***	−0.002	(−1.14)	–
Log—Price of Meat/Fish/Poultry	0.005	(2.53)	**	−0.002	(−1.45)	–	0.001	(0.42)	–	0.003	(2.54)	**
Log—Price of Pulses/Nuts/Others	−0.005	(−4.53)	***	−0.006	(−8.54)	***	−0.002	(−1.93)	*	−0.001	(−1.48)	–
Log—Price of Fruits	0.001	(0.66)	–	0.002	(2.45)	**	0.010	(7.87)	***	0.009	(12)	***
Log—Price of Vegetables	0.013	(3.94)	***	0.012	(5.55)	***	0.016	(4.91)	***	0.006	(3.53)	***

Log—Price of Cereals	0.009	(2.25)	**	0.009	(2.8)	***	−0.002	(−0.49)	–	−0.028	(−11.13)	***
Household Size	0.001	(2.41)	**	0.002	(10.78)	***	0.001	(3.59)	***	0.002	(16.48)	***
Proportion of Adult males in Household	0.035	(7.41)	***	0.026	(10.97)	***	0.024	(5.6)	***	0.020	(11.1)	***
Caste Dummy (ST)	−0.006	(−2.56)	**	0.002	(1.12)	–	−0.011	(−5.02)	***	−0.003	(−2.05)	**
Caste Dummy (Others)	−0.019	(−8.06)	***	−0.023	(−12.76)	***	−0.021	(−11.33)	***	−0.020	(−15.55)	***
Constant	0.861	(4.81)		2.662	(43.46)		−0.105	(−0.69)		2.427	(62.61)	
	Threshold Value: MPCE: Rs 16.0 Proportion of Calories from Cereals: 0.95						Threshold Value: MPCE: Rs 72.0 Proportion of Calories from Cereals: 0.85					

Source: Authors' calculations based on NSS (50th and 61st rounds).

Note: ***, **, and * refer to significance at the 1 per cent, 5 per cent, and 10 per cent level, respectively.

State Dummies are omitted and details will be furnished on request.

Among the poor, as in 1993, expenditure has a positive effect and its square has a negative effect on the calorie share. Both demographic variables (household size and proportion of adults) have significant positive effects. Both caste dummies (STs and others) have significant negative coefficients, implying lower calorie share than among the SCs. Food price effects are more varied than in 1993, while prices of milk and milk products and pulses/nuts/others have a negative effect (complements); by contrast, prices of vegetables, Vanaspati oil, eggs, and fruits have positive effects on calorie share (substitutes). The price of cereals has a negative impact on the share. Thus, calorie share is influenced not just by expenditure, demographic, and caste characteristics, but also by food prices.

Among the affluent, expenditure has a negative effect while its square has a positive effect. Both demographic variables (household size and proportion of adults) tend to raise the calorie share, while the caste variables (STs and others) are associated with lower shares relative to the SCs. While prices of cereals lower the calorie share, those of milk and milk products, Vanaspati oil, meat/fish/poultry, fruits, and vegetables raise it.

URBAN INDIA

The sample for urban India in 1993 yields results that are, in some respects, strikingly different from the rural results—especially the food price effects (Table 5.2).

Among the poor in urban India in 1993, both expenditure and its square have significant effects—positive and negative, respectively—on the calorie share. Proportion of adults has a significant positive effect while the caste dummies (STs and others) have negative effects (relative to the SCs). Three food price effects are significantly negative—milk and milk products, Vanaspati oil, and pulses/nuts/others—pointing to their complementarity to cereals. Prices of eggs and cereals have a positive impact on the calorie share from staples. Thus, the calorie share is sensitive to expenditure, demographic, and caste characteristics, and food prices.

Among the affluent, by contrast, expenditure and its square have significant effects (negative and positive, respectively). Demographic effects are significant too while the caste dummy for 'others' has a significant negative effect on the calorie share. Price of cereals has a negative effect, as also those of vanaspati oil, pulses/nuts/others,

TABLE 5.2 Regression Results: Urban India (1993 and 2004)

	Poor			Non-Poor			Poor			Non-Poor		
No. of observations	7000			28203			9813			26800		
Prob. > F	0.0000			0.0000			0.0000			0.0000		
	1993						2004					
Log MPCE	0.797	(11.63)	***	−0.488	(−30.82)	***	0.121	(3.95)	***	−0.452	(−30.43)	***
(Log MPCE)^2	−0.078	(−13.12)	***	0.024	(22.85)	***	−0.020	(−7.27)	***	0.023	(22.91)	***
Log—Price of Milk & Milk Products	−0.006	(−1.88)	*	0.017	(9.41)	***	0.002	(0.81)	–	0.004	(2.76)	***
Log—Price of Vanaspati Oil	−0.071	(−5.86)	***	−0.060	(−9.28)	***	0.044	(5.95)	***	0.013	(2.56)	**
Log—Price of Sugar	−0.009	(−1.1)	–	−0.001	(−0.17)	–	−0.025	(−3.49)	***	−0.049	(−11.08)	***
Log—Price of Eggs	0.006	(1.98)	**	0.008	(3.68)	***	0.017	(4.43)	***	0.012	(4.21)	***
Log—Price of Meat/ Fish/Poultry	−0.000	(−0.06)	–	0.006	(3)	***	0.004	(1.71)	*	0.010	(5.14)	***
Log—Price of Pulses/ Nuts/Others	−0.012	(−8.36)	***	−0.018	(−19.1)	***	−0.005	(−4.13)	***	−0.002	(−1.67)	*
Log—Price of Fruits	−0.003	(−1.45)	–	−0.002	(−1.03)	–	0.009	(4.73)	***	0.003	(2.19)	**
Log—Price of Vegetables	−0.007	(−1.62)	–	−0.007	(−3.06)	***	0.006	(1.64)	–	−0.003	(−1.16)	–
Log—Price of Cereals	0.015	(2.12)	**	−0.032	(−7.35)	***	−0.046	(−9.39)	***	−0.050	(−14.88)	***

(continued)

TABLE 5.2 Continued

	Poor			Non-Poor			Poor			Non-Poor		
	1993						2004					
Household Size	0.000	(0.38)	–	0.003	(9.79)	★★★	0.001	(3.45)	★★★	0.003	(10.99)	★★★
Proportion of Adult males in Household	0.036	(6.76)	★★★	0.051	(23.13)	★★★	0.033	(9)	★★★	0.028	(13.53)	★★★
Caste Dummy (ST)	−0.008	(−1.54)	–	0.001	(0.41)	–	−0.013	(−3.97)	★★★	−0.016	(−5.35)	★★★
Caste Dummy (Others)	−0.033	(−6.73)	★★★	−0.031	(−10.69)	★★★	−0.025	(−8.36)	★★★	−0.032	(−12.5)	★★★
Constant	−0.977	(−4.76)		2.999	(48.12)		0.590	(6.16)		2.733	(46.16)	
	Threshold Value: MPCE: Rs 166.4 Proportion of Calories from Cereals: 0.79						Threshold Value: MPCE: Rs 21.8 Proportion of Calories from Cereals: 0.88					

Source: Authors' calculations based on NSS (50th and 61st rounds).

Note: ★★★, ★★, and ★ refer to significance at the 1 per cent, 5 per cent, and 10 per cent level, respectively.

State Dummies are omitted and details will be furnished on request.

and vegetables. Price of milk/milk products, eggs, and meat/poultry/fish has a positive impact.

Let us now discuss the results for urban India in 2004 given in Table 5.2.

Among the poor, expenditure and its square are significant in determining the calorie share. Proportion of adults and household size have a positive effect while both caste dummies have negative effects (relative to the SCs). Prices of cereals, sugar, and of pulses/nuts/others lower this share, while those of vanaspati oil, eggs, meat/poultry/fish, vegetables, and fruits raise it. Food prices thus matter along with expenditure and other explanatory variables.

Among the affluent, expenditure has a negative effect, while its square has a positive effect on the calorie share. Demographic variables have positive effects while caste variables have negative effects on this share. All food prices other than those of vegetables have significant effects. Prices of cereals, pulses/nuts/others, and sugar have negative effects while those of milk and milk products, vanaspati oil, eggs, fruits, and meat/fish/poultry have positive effects.

For an assessment of relative importance of expenditure and price effects, their elasticities were computed. To avoid repetition, our comments are selective and brief.[12]

Expenditure elasticities for the poor in rural India remained stable over the period 1993–2004, at –0.14. By contrast, the elasticity (in absolute value) reduced in urban India (from over –0.20 to –0.17). Among the affluent, their (absolute) values fell more in urban India than in rural India. In both rural and urban India, and in both 1993 and 2004, the (absolute) expenditure elasticities were lower for the poor.

Confining to food price elasticities which had significant regression coefficients, an important finding is that while they vary between food commodities, across different sub-samples, and over time, they are substantially lower (in absolute value) than expenditure elasticities, implying that expenditure has a much larger influence on calorie shares (Table 5.3).

In sum, while these elasticities point to the more important role of expenditure in determining calorie share of cereals, they nevertheless corroborate that food prices matter too.

Estimates of Undernourished

To facilitate comparison of results obtained using Lowess (with expenditure) and robust regression (with expenditure, demographic, and caste

TABLE 5.3 Price and Expenditure Elasticities

	Rural 1993		Rural 2004		Urban 1993		Urban 2004	
	Poor	Non-Poor	Poor	Non-Poor	Poor	Non-Poor	Poor	Non-Poor
MPCE	−0.142*	−0.205*	−0.141*	−0.190*	−0.201*	−0.272*	−0.165*	−0.234*
Price of milk & milk products			−0.004*	0.010*	−0.008*	0.029*		0.007*
Price of vanaspati oil		−0.019*	0.043*	0.033*	−0.098*	−0.107*	0.062*	0.023*
Price of sugar	−0.014*			−0.041*			−0.034*	−0.087*
Price of eggs		0.006*	0.011*		0.009*	0.014*	0.024*	0.022*
Price of meat/fish/poultry	0.007*			0.005*		0.010*	0.005*	0.017*
Price of pulses/nuts/others	−0.006*	−0.009*	−0.003*		−0.017*	−0.032*	−0.007*	−0.003*
Price of fruits		0.004*	0.013*	0.014*			0.012*	0.005*
Price of vegetables	0.016*	0.017*	0.021*	0.009*		−0.013*		
Price of cereals	0.011*	0.013*		−0.043*	0.021*	−0.057*	−0.064*	−0.089*

Source: Authors' calculations based on NSS (50th and 61st rounds).

Note: * Elasticities of variables with significant regression coefficients have been reported.

characteristics, and food prices), various calorie share of cereals thresholds and implied estimates of undernourished are given below in Table 5.4. Graphical illustrations of the relationship between calorie share of cereals and MPCE, splicing together the results for the two subsets of the poor and affluent, are given in the Annexure.

The calorie thresholds obtained from Lowess are lower than those obtained from robust regressions, while expenditure thresholds are considerably higher. As a result, the estimates of undernourished vary greatly. Consider, for example, the estimates for rural India. The Lowess estimate is about 27 per cent, while the robust regression estimate for 1993 is 0.3 per cent. For 2004, the Lowess estimate is three times that of the robust regression estimate. Besides, while proportion of undernourished increases using robust regression estimates, it contrasts with a sharp reduction in Lowess estimates. Similarly, for urban India, the estimate of undernourished from Lowess is about twice that obtained from robust regression for 1993 and about thirty-five times that for 2004.

In sum, what our analysis points to is that the Jensen and Miller (2011) story is of limited interest and potentially misleading, principally because it confines variation in calorie share to a measure of wealth. The calorie and associated income thresholds are suspect as they are influenced by several other factors—especially food prices—that are omitted. Of particular interest is the finding that even the poor substitute in response to changes in food prices, and consequently the thresholds, change. Besides, the estimates of undernourished are vitiated by the failure to distinguish between those who are above the calorie threshold at extremely low expenditures and those with much higher expenditures. As these changed differently over the period 1993–2004, and arguably, call for different policies, the new measure has limited analytical and policy appeal.[13]

***

Decline in calorie intake—especially from cereals—across all expenditure classes during a period of accelerated economic growth is puzzling. Associated with the reduction in calorie intake is a related worry of a sharp rise in the proportion of calorie deprived, relative to widely used calorie norms. Many remain sceptical of this finding on the grounds that the calorie norms are no longer relevant because of two significant changes: (i) improvements in the social epidemiology of infectious disease, and (ii) lifestyle changes, including less strenuous activity patterns.

TABLE 5.4 Comparison of Calorie Share of Cereals Thresholds and Undernourished in India, 1993–2004*

Sample	Calorie Share of Cereals Threshold	Expenditure Threshold (Rs)	Below Expenditure Threshold but above Calorie Threshold (%)	Above Expenditure Threshold but above Calorie Threshold (%)	Total Undernourished (% Share of Population)
Rural 1993	0.95	16.0	0.00	0.32	0.32
	(0.80)	(200.3)	(2.64)	(24.72)	(27.36)
Rural 2004	0.85	72.0	0.00	5.23	5.23
	(0.80)	(244.7)	(3.43)	(12.64)	(16.07)
Urban 1993	0.79	166.4	0.07	7.69	7.76
	(0.75)	(270.4)	(1.21)	(13.37)	(14.58)
Urban 2004	0.88	21.8	0.00	0.24	0.24
	(0.75)	(270.4)	(1.04)	(7.56)	(8.60)

Source: Authors' calculations based on NSS (50th and 61st rounds).

Note: * Robust regression results are accompanied by Lowess results in parentheses.

Since no estimates are given of what these changes imply in terms of reduction of calorie 'requirements', measurement of undernutrition remains fraught with difficulties. As illustrated, even if a substantial reduction in calorie requirements is allowed for, the proportion of undernourished rises during the period 1993–2004. So the new measure proposed by Jensen and Miller (2011), dispensing with calorie norms and relying on a behavioural approach, seemed promising. Our analysis, however, raises serious doubts about the calorie share of cereals/staples threshold as the basis of measurement of undernutrition. First, although the theoretical rationale of this measure is consistent with the results obtained for China—in particular, a constrained utility maximization model with a penalty constraint that decreases as hunger diminishes—it is also consistent with a lexicographic preference for cereals/staples. The latter undermines the constrained utility maximization model. Second, absence of food prices in constructing the calorie share threshold flies in the face of substantial evidence, confirming substitution between food commodities even among the poor in response to changing prices. Indeed, assuming away of their taste for variety undermines the behavioural approach. Third, experiments with an expanded specification, incorporating not just expenditure but also demographic and caste characteristics, and food prices for various commodities imply large differences in proportions of undernourished both in the same year and over time.

In any case, the policy implications are worrying as the important role of food price stabilization in mitigating undernutrition is overlooked. While the PDS has considerable potential, its benefits are limited by high transaction costs for the poor. Universalization of the food subsidy would be not just enormously wasteful, but also fiscally unsustainable.

In conclusion, not just predictive accuracy of the new measure proposed, but also its descriptive richness leave much to be desired. From a policy perspective, careful attention must be given to livelihood expansion and food price stabilization.

ANNEXURE

Graphical Illustrations

Figure 5A.1 gives graphs of calorie share of food grains with respect to monthly per capita expenditure (MPCE) in rural and urban India in 1993 and 2004, based on robust regressions.

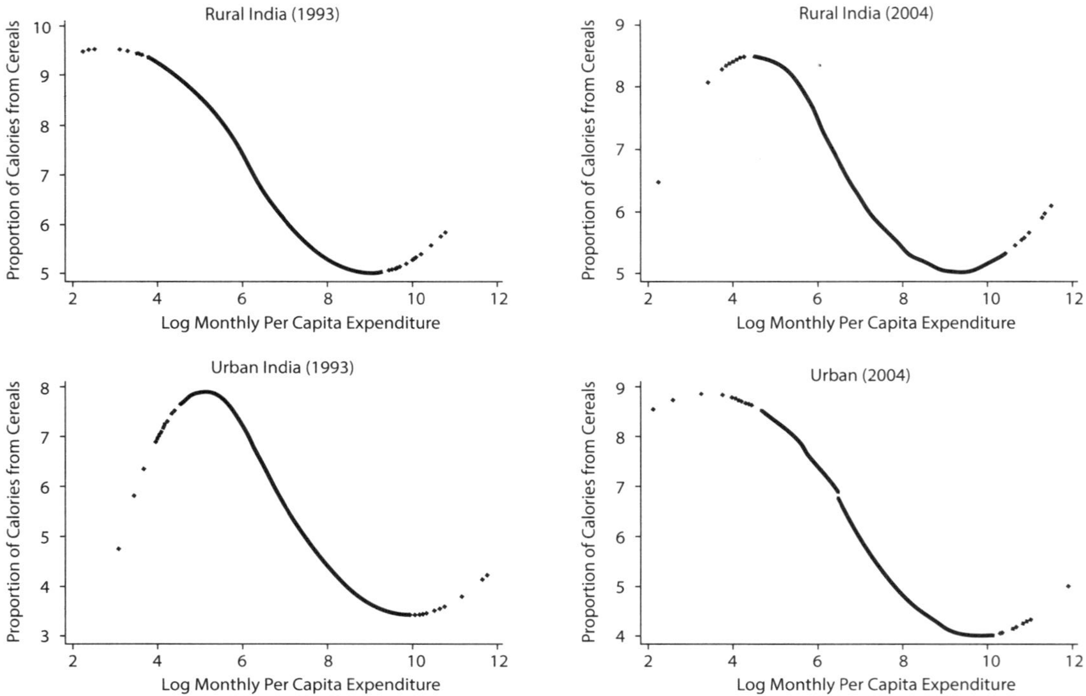

FIGURE 5A.1 Calorie Share of Food Grains by Monthly Per Capita Expenditure in Rural and Urban India, 1993–2004.

Source: NSS 50th and 61st rounds.

NOTES

1. Refer to Chapter 2 for a discussion on Deaton and Dréze's (2009) findings on decline in calorie intakes and the explanation offered. We also offer a demand based explanation of this decline in Chapter 2.
2. For an exposition, see FAO's SOFI (2012), and for an influential critique, see Srinivasan (1992). The issue of calorie norms, however, remains largely unresolved.
3. For an insightful exposition, see Behrman and Deolalikar (1989). For illustrative results with India's data, see Jha *et al.* (2009b).
4. A search in the neighbourhood of where a switch seems to occur helps identify the threshold.
5. In rural India in 1993, cereals accounted for about 71 per cent of total calories, while in 2004, the corresponding share dropped to about 68 per cent (Gaiha *et al.* 2010, 2012).
6. The utility function u (x_1, x_2) is a standard utility function minus a penalty function, f (.), maximized subject to a wealth/budget constraint. u (.) is assumed to be homothetic. This implies that the marginal rate of substitution between x_1 and x_2 depends only on their ratio, x_1/x_2. f (.) represents a penalty function that is decreasing and convex. Letting $z=c_1x_1+c_2x_2-s$, where x_1 and x_2 are two food commodities, c_1 and c_2 denote their calorie content, and s is a constant that captures subsistence calories, it is further assumed that f'(z) increases to 0 as z increases above 0 and decreases to negative infinity as z decreases below 0. When the consumer is sufficiently wealthy, f'(z) will approach 0, and so the consumer behaves approximately as if he maximizes u(x) subject to the budget constraint. However, at low wealth, the consumer finds it difficult to afford a bundle with z>0, and behaves approximately as if he maximizes calories subject to the budget constraint (Jensen and Miller 2011).
7. Nine commodities are distinguished, comprising cereals, milk and milk products, vanaspati oil, sugar, eggs, meat/fish and poultry, pulses/nuts/dry fruits, fruits, and vegetables. For details of their calorie content, see Gaiha *et al.* (2010).
8. Briefly, Lowess is used for locally weighted scatterplot smoothing. The smoothed values are obtained by running a regression of *yvar* on *xvar*, using only the data (x_i, y_i) and a small amount of the data near this point. The regression is weighted so that the central point (x_i, y_i) gets the highest weight and points that are farther away (based on the distance $|x_j - x_i|$) receive less weight. The estimated regression line is then used to predict the smoothed value of $\hat{y}_i$ for y_i only. This procedure is repeated to obtain the remaining smoothed values. Thus a separate weighted regression is performed for every point in the data. For a more detailed but intuitive exposition, see Deaton (1995).

9. For a recent analysis of dietary transition in India driven by growth of income and urbanization, food prices, and expansion of the middle class, see Kaicker *et al.* (2011).

10. The poverty cut-off point for rural India is Rs 358 and for urban India Rs 540.

11. For expositional convenience, and given a monotonic relationship between expenditure and its logarithmic transformation, expenditure is synonymous with its log.

12. All elasticity comparisons are in terms of absolute values unless stated otherwise.

13. Why descriptive richness of an explanation matters and not just its predictive accuracy was persuasively argued by Sen (2005).

6 Poverty Nutrition Traps in Rural India*

Raghbendra Jha, Raghav Gaiha, and Anurag Sharma

UNICEF (2006) has noted that as many as 57 million children under the age of five are undernourished in India. While this is an immediate area of concern since reducing undernutrition forms one of the Millennium Development Goals, another important concern is whether such undernutrition impacts labour productivity, thus reducing the possibility that earnings from the labour market could be used to reduce undernutrition. World Bank (2006) estimates that India lost $2.5 billion in 2005 because of reduced productivity from undernutrition.

The effect of nutritional intake on labour productivity and wage rates has been an important area of research for health economists and nutritionists for some time. This found initial expression in the form of the efficiency wage hypothesis developed by Leibenstein (1957) and Mazumdar (1959), and was formalized and extended by Mirrlees (1975), Dasgupta and Ray (1986, 1987), and Dasgupta (1993, 1997), among others. Early surveys include Bliss and Stern (1978a, 1978b), and Binswanger and Rosenzweig (1984). More recent critiques include Srinivasan (1994), and Banerjee and Duflo (2011), among others. The efficiency wage hypothesis postulated that in developing countries, particularly at low levels of nutrition, workers are physically incapable of doing hard manual labour. Hence their productivity is low, which then

* Reprinted from *World Development*, vol. 37, no. 5, R. Jha, R. Gaiha, and A. Sharma, 'Calorie and Macronutrient Deprivation and Poverty Nutrition Traps in Rural India', pp. 982–91, May 2009, with permission from Elsevier Limited.

implies that they get low wages, have low purchasing power, and therefore, low levels of nutrition, completing a vicious cycle of deprivation. As these workers are unable to save very much, their assets—both physical and human—are minimal. This reduces their chances of escaping the poverty nutrition trap (PNT).[1]

There is substantial literature on empirically testing for the existence of PNT (Strauss and Thomas 1998). Thomas and Strauss (1997), for example, investigate the impact of four indicators of health (height, body mass index, per capita calorie intake, and per capita protein intake) on wages of workers in urban Brazil. They discover that even after accounting for endogeneity issues and controlling for education and other dimensions of health, these four indicators have significant positive effects on wages. The effect of the nutritional variables—per capita calorie intake and per capita protein intake—was higher at low levels of nutrition. In contrast, Deolalikar (1988) finds in a (panel fixed effects) joint regression of the wage equation and farm production in rural South India that calorie intake does not affect either, but a measure of weight-for-height does. He concludes that calorie intake does not affect wages or productivity, indicating that the human body can adapt to short-run shortfalls in calorie intake. However, the fact that weight-for-height affects wages and productivity indicates that undernutrition is an important determinant of productivity and wages. Swamy (1997) argues that there is only weak support for the efficiency wage hypothesis in the data set on India that he worked with since a cut in the wage rate would lower the efficiency cost of labour without reducing productivity. However, this analysis is based on very small sample sizes and does not involve a formal test of the efficiency wage hypotheses, as it is confined to computing the cost per efficiency unit of labour.

Furthermore, the PNT argument has often been motivated in terms of calorie deficiency. It has also been argued that, to the extent that deficiencies of other nutrients are correlated with calorie deficiency, it may not be necessary to model the PNT in terms of nutrients other than calories. However, if deprivation in terms of other nutrients is higher than that for calories, and different categories of workers are affected by calorie deprivation and other nutrient deprivation, a modelling of the PNT in terms of other nutrients is still relevant. Furthermore, micronutrient deficiency has independent deleterious effects on health and productivity. Thus Barrett (2002) indicates that micronutrient deficiency directly reduces cognitive and physical activity, and hence, labour productivity. Besides, such deficiency indirectly reduces labour productivity by increasing susceptibility to diseases and infections. Horton and Ross (2003) show that iron deficiency in developing countries is related to a variety of functional consequences with economic implications such as mental impairment in children, and low work productivity in adults. Hence, it is important to examine the productivity effects—in particular, the PNT implications of micronutrient deficiency in addition to calorie deficiency—on which most of the literature has concentrated.[2]

A significant gap in the extant literature on India is the neglect of the impact of micronutrient deprivation on labour productivity—including the possibility of the existence of a PNT with respect to micronutrients. In an important contribution, Weinberger (2003) discusses the impact of iron deficiency on labour productivity in rural India, but does not model the impact of micronutrient deficiency on PNT. To the best of our knowledge there does not exist any study quantifying the importance of micronutrient deficiency in the formation of PNT. The present analysis attempts to fill this gap. We test for the existence of a PNT in the case of calories and four key micronutrients[3]—carotene, iron, riboflavin, and thiamine—for three categories of wages (sowing, harvesting, and other), and for male and female workers separately.

The scheme of this chapter is as follows: it undertakes the analysis of PNT, discusses the data, demonstrates the estimation methodology, and finally, presents the results of the estimation.

PNTs

Why poverty and undernutrition persist in developing countries has been subjected to critical scrutiny in important recent contributions (Dasgupta and Ray 1986, 1987; Dasgupta 1997, 2009; Svedberg 2000).

Let us first consider intuitively the model(s) proposed by Dasgupta.[4] Two assumptions are invoked: (i) maintenance requirement is a large fraction of total energy expenditure (60–75 per cent goes towards maintenance and the remaining 25–40 per cent is spent on 'discretionary' activities—work and leisure); and (ii) at levels of energy intake exceeding maintenance requirement, there are diminishing gains in productivity from further increases in consumption. Of the two, the first assumption is crucial for understanding why a society's poverty causes stark inequality in striking contrast to a common presumption that inequality causes poverty.

Let us consider a private ownership agrarian economy with a large number of assetless people relative to the aggregate wealth of the economy. Two further assumptions are used here: (i) the economy in the aggregate is poor; and (ii) the distribution of assets is unequal. For simplicity, all are identical in nutritional status. Agricultural market is characterized by long-term contracts. The only alternative to agricultural employment is to live off common property resources (for example, forest products)—an inferior option.

A person either works in agriculture or lives off the commons. Imagine that the efficient productivity level of a landless agricultural worker is achieved at an energy intake that is greater than the amount available from the commons. Living off the commons thus results in a steady deterioration in nutritional status. Under these assumptions, the agricultural labour market does not clear. Or, there is no wage rate at which demand for labour equals its supply. So there is rationing, and a fraction of the landless find employment in agriculture, while the remaining live off the commons. Those employed receive a wage rate equal to the wage at which efficient productivity is attained (efficient wage hypothesis). The unemployed cannot undercut the employed as it would make them less attractive as workers. Thus different classes emerge from a homogeneous group.[5]

Various critiques rely on related evidence and their implications.

- No more than 15–20 per cent of a casual agricultural labourer's wage is needed to break out of the PNT.
- There is a wide range of calorie intake responses to higher expenditure (Behrman and Deolalikar 1987; Subramanian and Deaton 1996), but in no case it is unity.
- The implication that there is budgetary slack among the poor is then used to reject the PNT model (Srinivasan 1994; Strauss and Thomas 1995; Subramanian and Deaton 1996).
- Banerjee and Duflo (2011) point out that in reality the poor do not spend their money solely on high calorie, cheap food, but on luxury food and entertainment. This discrepancy is cited as evidence that a

nutrition-base poverty trap does not exist. Dasgupta (1997, 2009), however, rejects the budget slack argument by pointing out that the poor have other priorities too—support for other family members, contingencies, and other nutrients' requirements.

Another interesting model, but with a somewhat broader objective, is formulated in Svedberg (2000). It focuses on the behaviour of nutritionally constrained individuals who face given prices in which they can choose their workload. A distinction is made between the biological production function that converts the energy in food into muscular activity, and the economical production function that turns this muscular activity into work which earns an income. Job-specific wages are exogenously determined by aggregate demand and supply in which the individual works (being unrelated to the nutritional status of the individual). The central issue is not unemployment, but how a poor individual's economic and biological behaviour is affected by energy entering as an input in the labour production function.

For an individual engaged in a given work activity, an exogenous increase in his wage (or price of the product) makes him increase his work activity and body weight, and thus his calorie intake/expenditure. Or, the association between calorie intake and income is positive. Alternatively, income or food in kind support could also reduce calorie intake if (s)he has disutility of effort. Due to inter-individual differences in the work activities (more or less physically demanding) and in biological characteristics, higher incomes are associated with lower calorie intake (or body weight). A reason is that well-paid jobs are often less physically demanding than low-paid manual jobs. But there is no causality as both income and nutrition are endogenous.[6]

While both the Dasgupta and Svedberg models seek to throw light on the persistence of undernutrition and poverty, there are some striking differences in the determination of agricultural wage rate, labour market equilibrium, and dynamics of nutrition-poverty linkages. The latter, for example, is static, and does not illuminate the dynamic pathways through which the individual adjusts his work effort, calorie intake, and body weight in the face of exogenous shocks. Nor does it offer insights into intra-household inequality. So, despite its somewhat narrow focus, we have chosen the Dasgupta model(s) for empirical validation.

DATA AND METHODOLOGY

The data used in this paper came from the National Council for Applied Economic Research (NCAER). The data were collected through a multi-purpose household survey, designed and conducted by the NCAER. This survey was spread over six months, from January to June, 1994.[7] The data were collected using varied reference periods based on some conventional rules. For example, to estimate household income in rural agricultural households, cultivation and output figures used refer to the previous agricultural year. Similarly, to estimate short duration morbidity, occurrence of sickness during the preceding thirty days was recorded, but for major morbidity, the reference period was the previous year.

A multi-stage sample design was chosen, in light of cost and time considerations, operational feasibility, and precision of the estimates. In each of the sixteen states covered, the districts were cross-classified by income from agriculture and rural female literacy rate to form homogeneous strata in terms of these two variables. From each of these strata, a pre-assigned number of districts, depending on the size of the stratum, were selected with probability proportional to the rural population in the district. Given the list of villages in the sample districts in the 1991 Census records, a pre-assigned number of villages were then selected linear systematically after arranging the villages in a *tehsil* (an administrative block), alternately in ascending and descending order of rural female literacy. The households in the sample villages were listed along with information such as religion, caste, major sources of income, cultivable land, and other social and demographic characteristics, as well as the occupation of the head of the household. Sample households from each of the strata so formed were selected linear systematically. Thus a total sample of 35,130 households spread over 1,765 villages and 195 districts in sixteen states was covered in the survey.

We had data on actual rainfall for 1994 and average rainfall for 69 of the 76 agro-climatic zones in the country, and both were needed to construct our rainfall index. Our dataset is further restricted by the non-availability of wage data for as many as 9,838 households. We also needed food price data at the village level since these are crucially required as instruments for the estimation. These data were not available for a major chunk of the remaining households. The remaining data comprised information on 6,594 households. Our analysis, therefore, covers this set of households.

A detailed commodity classification was used, together with careful measurement of physical quantities of food items consumed. In addition, data on household expenditure on these items were canvassed. Food intake was converted into nutrients consumed using the conversion factors (Gopalan *et al.* 1971; ICMR 1990)—these are the most detailed and widely used conversion factors in India and have been used by a number of authors to convert food intake into their nutritional equivalents. Also collected are data on expenditures on various items. We divide expenditure by quantity to obtain estimates of unit price, following Deaton and Tarozzi (2000). These unit prices/values are aggregated at village level to average out extreme values as well as to remove their endogeneity.

The NCAER survey combines a detailed classification of food commodities with a careful measurement of physical quantities consumed. The conversion of food items consumed into nutrient intakes is thus reliable.

The wage data used (available on a daily basis) are those for harvesting, sowing, and other occupations for male and female workers separately. Table 6.1 shows the distribution of male and female workers over the various occupational categories in these households. Mean wage rates per day for specific tasks were: Male Sowing (Rs 12.26), Male Harvesting (Rs 17.56), Male Other (Rs 15.28), Female Sowing (Rs 7.86), Female Harvesting (Rs 12.06), and Female Other (Rs 7.94).[8]

Any empirical strategy to estimate the PNT must deal with the mutual endogeneity of wage and nutrition. We have used the well-known Heckman self-selection procedure. The problem of sample selection arises when the data in the survey are incidentally truncated or non-randomly selected (Greene 2003).[9] Our model determining wage nutrition relationship contains the following main regression equation:

$$Y_i = \beta' X_i + \varepsilon_i \tag{1}$$

where Y_i is the wage rate and X_i is a vector comprising the nutrition and other household characteristics. The model may imply a wage rate

TABLE 6.1 Number of Male and Female Workers in Different Occupational Categories

Employment Category	No. of Male Workers	No. of Female Workers
Sowing	2151	1800
Harvesting	2717	2201
Other	2660	1922

Source: Authors' computations.

for all the individuals, but we observe it only for those who are actually employed. Hence, the model is truncated as the sample is selected on the basis of wages (in the agricultural sector).

Formally, the wages are observed only if:

$$Z_i\star = \gamma' W_i + u_i \tag{2}$$

W_i are independent variables that contribute to the employment probability of an individual. W_i may or may not overlap with the X_i.

Equation (2) is the selection equation. The sample rule thus becomes that $W_i\star$ (the wage rate) is observed only when $Z_i\star > 0$ (or the person under consideration is employed in the agricultural sector).

Our choice of variables for the two stages of the estimation is justified as follows. In the selection equation, higher rainfall increases the intensity of agricultural activity, and hence, employment. In addition, we employ a number of household characteristics that are commonly used in the literature (for example, age of household head and its square, gender of household head, number of adult males and females in the household, land possessed by the household and its square, and the social group—Scheduled Castes (SCs) or Scheduled Tribes (STs)—to which the household belongs). In addition, we control for state level effects such as economic backwardness (Bihar, Madhya Pradesh, Rajasthan, and Uttar Pradesh, abbreviated as BIMARU) or whether they are coastal, through dummy variables. These variables have implications for job-search (job search is less costly with better infrastructure and easier access to labour markets), and farm and non-farm employment opportunities.

For the second stage estimation, the wage rates are modelled as a function of predicted nutrient intake and its square (separately for each regression), rainfall, and all other household characteristics used in the first stage. The inclusion of the predicted nutrient and its square are motivated by the PNT analysis; rainfall will affect agricultural output, and hence agricultural wages and household characteristics are included because these might independently affect the wage earned (for example, reservation wage would vary with the amount of land possessed, and inversely with SC/ST affiliation). Dummy variables for the traditionally less well-off states (BIMARU) and coastal states, such as Maharashtra, Karnataka, and Tamil Nadu, are included because these may have state level effects on the agricultural wage. In addition, prices for four food groups, pulses, *gur*/sugar, edible oil, and milk, are included. These are the only food groups for which complete data covering the whole sample are available. These food items cover the most important categories of foods: pulses are consumed as a major food item, gur/sugar and edible oil are intermediates, and milk is a relative luxury for the poor.

RESULTS

The case for analysing PNT with respect to micronutrients gathers additional relevance if it places emphasis on both direct and indirect effects of food prices on agricultural wages. The indirect effect is through the nutrient intake (Behrman and Deolaikar 1990; Lakdawala *et al.* 2005; Pitt and Rosenzweig 1986), whereas the direct effect is through labour market responses emanating from changes in the food market (Bardhan 1984; Barrett and Dorosh 1996; Datt and Olmsted 2004; Gaiha 1995; Ravallion 1990; Sah and Stiglitz 1987). We include the nutritional status and food prices in the wage equation to capture both types of effects. Level of deprivation with respect to micronutrients is greater than that for calories, the traditional nutrient used in the analysis of PNT. In Table 6.2 we depict the deficiency with respect to calories and the selected four micronutrients.

The nutritional intake at household level was converted into per capita male equivalent. This was then compared to male equivalent recommended dietary allowances (RDA) cut-offs to determine nutritional deficiency. The per cent of households experiencing a deficiency with respect to calories is lower than that for all other nutrients except thiamine. In view of the fact that micronutrient deficiency affects

TABLE 6.2 Nutrient Deficiency: Summary Statistics

Micronutrient	Percentage of Households Deficient in★★★	Minimum Recommended Daily Allowance★★
Energy★	77.3	2800 (Calories)
Iron	77.6	20 (mg.)
Carotene	100	2000 (IU.)
Thiamine★	42.5	1.4 (mg.)
Riboflavin★	90.24	1.5 (mg.)

Source: Authors' calculations based on IHDS, 1994.

Notes: ★ Daily allowance for moderate work.

★★ Allowance for Indians based on recommendations by Nutrition Expert Groups (Table 2), Gopalan *et al.* (1971) and ICMR (1990). For example, it is recorded that 100g of par-boiled, hand-pounded rice yields 349 calories of energy, 10 mg of calcium, 2.8mg of iron, and 9μg of carotene.

★★★ Deficiency computed in terms of adult male equivalent size of household. The use of per capita food intake accounts for the number of persons taking part in the meals, but not the composition of the household in terms of sex, age, and body size. This may be misleading as a welfare indicator as food intake is influenced by food energy requirements, which are determined primarily by sex and age, in addition to other factors such as activity level. For example, a household including young children is expected to have a lower energy intake than a household consisting of only adults, because children's energy requirements, and consequently their food needs, are lower than those of adults. The adult male equivalence scale was developed to provide an expression of household food intake that accounts for the composition of the household and allows the direct comparison of food or energy intakes of households of different sizes and compositions. For details of how these scales are constructed, see Lanjouw and Ravallion (1995); Weisell and Claude Dop (2012).

labour productivity, it can be surmised that there is a strong case for studying the PNT for nutrients other than calories as well.

PNT, that is, the existence of a bi-directional relationship between wages and nutritional intake, represents a standard problem of endogeneity in econometric terms: if wages affect nutrition and nutrition affects wages, they are both endogenous to the system. An econometric test which confirms endogeneity implies existence of PNT. We perform the Durbin-Wu-Hausman test which comprises a test for endogeneity in a regression estimated via instrumental variables (IV), the null hypothesis for which states that an ordinary least squares (OLS) estimator of the same equation would yield consistent estimates; that is, any endogeneity among the regressors would not have deleterious effects on OLS estimates. Once an endogenous relationship between wages and nutritional intake (PNT) is established, the next issue is choice of model specification (whether wage should be a function of nutritional intake or vice versa). This is required to estimate elasticities and marginal effects. We have chosen a specification where wages are a function of nutritional intake (which is instrumented) mainly for two reasons: (i) our focus is on analysing the impact of policies to improve nutritional intake on agricultural wages, and (ii) given the nature of our dataset, it is easier to find potential instruments for nutritional intake than wages. Thus we have instrumented nutrient intake and its squared value. Religion dummies are used as identifying instruments for nutritional intake. Dietary behaviour (which implicitly captures health effects) is controlled in the first stage predictive equations of nutrients. This is done by incorporating religion dummies. In India, religious practices are crucial to dietary behaviour. Buddhists, Jains, and most sub-castes of Hindus follow a strict vegetarian diet. The extant literature on dietary behaviour in India has shown that Muslims and Christians tended to have similar dietary intakes. The Hindus have the lowest nutrient intake for protein, fat, calories, and calcium. Six dummy variables are generated for religion with Hindu as the base case. All dummy variables are significant and positive for each nutrient, confirming that Hindus have lower nutrient intake compared to other religious groups. In addition to religion dummies, all other exogenous variables are automatically included as instruments to maximize efficiency of IV estimation.

Diagnostics for first stage regressions, in particular the robust F-test for predictive equations of each nutrient instrumented, not reported here to save space, indicate that coefficients in first stage regressions are jointly significant for all categories of nutrients.

Table 6.3 reports the coefficient on the respective per capita nutrient in the wage equations and the associated Hausman statistic. Under the null, the Hausman statistic is distributed as Chi-squared with 'm' degrees of freedom, where 'm' is the number of regressors specified as endogenous in the original instrumental variables regression. The corresponding 'p' values show that the null is rejected in all the cases,

TABLE 6.3 Main Results Demonstrating Existence of PNT

Nutrient Category	Coefficient on Per Capita Nutrient	Hausman Test (chi2 statistic) for Endogeneity
Calories (calories/day)		
Female Sowing	0.017	61.35
	(0.001)	(0.001)
Female Harvesting	0.013	28.11
	(0.001)	(0.005)
Carotene (microgram/day)		
Male Harvesting	0.042	29.99
	(0.009)	(0.001)
Iron (milligram/day)		
Female Harvesting	0.406	20.17
	(0.001)	(0.043)
Male Harvesting	0.598	23.17
	(0.001)	(0.016)
Riboflavin (milligram/day)		
Female Harvesting	19.68	27.78
	(0.001)	(0.007)
Female Sowing	7.95	30.90
	(0.08)	(0.001)
Male Harvesting	16.57	15.53
	(0.022)	(0.015)
Thiamine (milligram/day)		
Female Harvesting	6.99	26.60
	(0.001)	(0.005)
Female Sowing	4.06	41.10
	(0.019)	(0.001)

Source: Authors' calculations based on IHDS, 1994.
Note: *P* values in parentheses.

or OLS is inconsistent and instrumental variables techniques are required. This test also confirms the validity of our instrumental variable approach, and establishes the existence of PNT in these cases.

Detailed results (including the selection equation) for the ten cases where the PNT is found to exist are shown in Table 6.4. This table shows the impact of respective per capita consumption of nutrient (and its square) for the case of each nutrient and other variables used in the regression along with results on the Heckman selection equation. The latter are based on a probit and shown in the bottom panel.

The Heckman estimation of the PNT model shows that PNT exists in one-third (that is, ten) of the thirty cases. It exists for female harvest wage and female sowing wage for calories. In the case of carotene, male workers engaged in harvesting are subject to the PNT, whereas both male and female workers engaged in harvesting are subject to PNT in the case of iron. In the case of riboflavin, female workers engaged in harvesting and sowing and male workers engaged in harvesting are subject to PNT, and in the case of thiamine, female workers engaged in harvesting and sowing are subject to PNT. In all these cases, the coefficients of the predicted nutrient and its square are strongly significant and have the right signs, thus indicating the presence of PNT in these cases. Since harvesting is more physically demanding than sowing, there is higher incidence of PNT in harvesting.

It should be noted that, whereas the PNT holds for calories only in the cases of female sowing and female harvesting wages, it holds for males in the case of male harvesting wages (carotene, iron, and riboflavin). Furthermore, for females PNT holds in respect of harvest and sowing wages for calories, thiamine, and riboflavin, but PNT does not exist for females in the case of carotene, and exists only for harvesting wages in the case of iron. Hence, an analysis which concentrates exclusively on energy intake may present an incomplete picture of the existence of PNT.

In the selection equation results (bottom of Table 6.4), rainfall is positive and significant at about the 10 per cent level. Neither the age of the head of the household, nor its square are significant. A larger number of adult males in the household has a significant negative effect, probably because adult males are substitutes for females in agricultural employment. A larger number of adult females in the household has a significant positive effect as this increases the number of workers available for working in agricultural activity. Hence adult females are complements, since one or two could handle household chores. It is well-known that the share of households belonging to disadvantaged groups (SCs and STs in particular) is disproportionately higher among the poor. Hence this variable is associated with a significant positive

TABLE 6.4 Results on Estimation of PNT Equations

Explanatory Variables	Calories, Female Sowing	Calories, Female Harvesting	Carotene, Male Harvesting	Iron, Female Harvesting	Iron, Male Harvesting	Riboflavin, Female Harvesting	Riboflavin, Female Sowing	Riboflavin, Male Harvesting	Thiamine, Female Harvesting	Thiamine, Female Sowing
Diagnostics	Waldchi 2(23) = 1175.47 Prob > chi2 = 0	Waldchi 2(23) = 1313.11 Prob > chi2 = 0	Waldchi 2(23) = 855.78 Prob > chi2 = 0	Waldchi 2(23) = 1307.95 Prob > chi2 = 0	Waldchi 2(23) = 857.62 Prob > chi2 = 0	Waldchi 2(23) = 1315.04 Prob > chi2 = 0	Waldchi 2(23) = 1163.96 Prob > chi2 = 0	Waldchi 2(23) = 855.85 Prob > chi2 = 0	Waldchi 2(23) = 1313 Prob > chi2 = 0	Waldchi 2(23) = 1161.76 Prob > chi2 = 0
Bimaru dummy	−5.8**	−8.3**	−4.5 **	−9.75**	−5.85**	−8.69**	−6.25**	−5.02**	−9.05 **	−6.71**
Coastal dummy	3.22**	3.2**	8.5**	4.09**	6.15**	4.85**	4.59**	7.75**	4.73**	4.51**
Predicted nutrient per capita	0.017**	0.013**	0.04*	0.4**	0.59**	19.68**	7.95**	16.57**	6.99**	4.06**
Predicted nutrient per capita square	−3.39E-06**	−2.13E-06**	−3.6E-05	−0.001	−0.0019	−3.1**	−2.65**	−1.01	−0.37**	−0.38**
Price of pulses	−0.06	−0.19**	−0.09	−0.15**	−0.08	−0.32**	−0.21**	−0.11	−0.27**	−0.16**
Price of gur/sugar	0.10	−0.27*	−0.75**	0.07	−1.01**	−0.46**	0.02	−0.99 **	−0.34*	0.09
Price of oil	−0.08**	0.068**	0.07**	0.05**	0.14**	0.014	−0.09**	0.096**	0.026	−0.1**
Price of Milk	−0.07**	−0.07**	−0.21**	−0.1**	−0.22**	−0.07**	−0.05*	−0.21**	−0.07**	−0.06**
Age of household head	0.18**	0.05	−0.19	−0.008	−0.28**	0.029	0.11*	−0.26**	0.013	0.08

Age of household head square	−0.002**	−0.0009	0.002	−0.0002	0.002**	−0.0008	−0.001**	0.002**	−0.0006	−0.001*
Number of adult males in household	−0.74**	−1.44**	−0.33	−1.53**	−0.75**	−1.32**	−0.57**	−0.47	−1.28**	−0.59**
Number of adult females in household	0.91**	1.33**	−0.35	1.32**	−0.6	2.14**	1.54**	−0.06	2.03**	1.56**
Household size	−0.53**	0.067	0.16	0.28	0.71**	−0.45**	−0.82**	0.23	−0.35*	−0.77**
SC/ST Dummy	4.99**	2.48**	3.45**	1.5**	4.24**	3.53**	5.09**	4.18**	3.13**	5.06**
Rainfall Index	−0.002 **	0.002**	−0.004**	0.002**	−0.003**	0.001**	−0.002**	−0.004**	0.002**	−0.002**
Constant	−7.22	0.55	23.65	5.35	17.93	17.7	13.21	24.65	14.79	10.629
Mills Lambda	0.87	−0.58	5.95**	−0.13	5.96**	−0.93	1.25	6.01**	−0.57	1.12
Rho	0.087	−0.049	0.36	−0.011	0.36	−0.079	0.12	0.36	−0.048	0.11
Sigma	10.02	11.75	16.47	11.75	16.47	11.76	10.05	16.48	11.75	10.05
Selection Equation	0.28 constant − 0.03 Age of household head + 2.98E-05 Age of household head squared − 0.03** Number of adult males in household + 0.05** number of adult females in household + 0.49** SC/ST dummy − 0.004** Area of land owned − 6.04E-08 Area of land owned squared + 8.92E-05* Rainfall index + 4.84E-06** Landowned × rain + 0.3** Bimaru dummy + 1.00** Coastal dummy + 0.24** Female household head dummy									

Source: Authors' calculations based on IHDS, 1994.

Note: **= significant at 5 per cent or less, *= significant at between 5 per cent and 10 per cent, remaining coefficients are insignificant.

impact on opting for agricultural activity. Consistent with this, since BIMARU states have higher than average incidence of poverty, households in such states show a greater tendency to opt for agricultural employment. Coastal states experience less uncertainty about rainfall, and hence have greater intensity of agricultural activity, *ceteris paribus*. Thus, this variable has a positive and significant coefficient in the selection equation. Finally, the share of female-headed households in the rural poor is in excess of their proportion in the population of households. Hence female-headed households show greater proclivity to engage in agricultural activity, and this variable has a positive and significant effect on the selection equation.

In the wage equation for sowing, rainfall has a negative and significant effect, reflecting the possibility that higher rainfall reduces the need for re-sowing, and hence lowers wages. Higher rainfall raises harvest prospects, and since female harvest wages are lower than male harvest wages, more females are employed and their wages go up. Commensurately, fewer males are employed for harvesting and male harvesting wages go down. The BIMARU dummy has a negative sign indicating that wages in such states are lower, relative to other states—particularly the more prosperous coastal states, the dummy for which has, in accordance with this argument, a positive and significant sign. Higher prices indicate lower availability of nutrients, *ceteris paribus*. Hence, in agreement with earlier studies (Bardhan 1984; Gaiha 1995; Ravallion 1990), higher food prices are typically associated with a negative and significant sign in the wage equations. The impact of age of head and its square varies over the various wage equations. Female wage rates drop as the number of adult males in the household rises, presumably because, *ceteris paribus*, more males are available for agricultural work (as noted earlier, because of the substitutability between males and females). The impact of the number of males on male wage rates is, however, not significant because some of them might migrate to non-agricultural work. Households with more adult females will have more female workers available for working in agricultural occupations, hence female wages rise. The number of adult females does not have a significant impact on male wage rates, since some of the males might migrate. The effect of household size varies over the wage and gender categories. Since SCs and STs constitute a disproportionately higher share of the poor, such households have higher number of agricultural labourers so that wage rates are higher, *ceteris paribus*, as our results indicate.[10]

In all these cases, the signs of the coefficients of predicted value of the nutrient and its square (say, the coefficients of predicted calorie per capita and its square) support the hypothesis that agricultural wages are non-linear functions of the respective nutrient intakes of workers, and also confirm the existence of PNT. In view of this, it becomes necessary to calculate the marginal effects of nutrients on wages. If these are positive and significant, then augmenting nutrient intake would help increase rural wages and, since agricultural workers are disproportionately represented in the rural poor, reduce rural poverty as well. This is an important implication for policy purposes.

The marginal effects are significant for all but one of the micronutrients and wage categories, and indicate that a policy to increase nutritional intake among the malnourished population can lead to increase in their wage earnings. This underlines the importance of a policy to provide direct nutritional supplements to the nutritionally deprived. The elasticities of wages (female sowing and harvesting) with respect to calories are relatively high; followed by those (female harvesting and male harvesting) with respect to iron; and then those (female harvesting) with respect to riboflavin and thiamine (female harvesting and female sowing).[11]

***

The possibility that when workers have inadequate intakes of energy and micronutrients, they may not be able to exert sufficient effort so that their wages remain low, which then leads to further poor nutritional outcomes, has been known in the literature for long. Several authors have tried to empirically test for the existence of this trap, but none have been able to establish unambiguously that this holds for a subset of the working population and not the whole, and there has been no attempt to do so for micronutrients. Further, the extant literature also has not explored the existence of PNT by gender and occupation.

Our analysis has attempted to quantify and formally test for the presence of PNT in rural India. It outlines a methodology that can identify the impact of nutrients' consumption on wage rates, even in the presence of mutual endogeneity. As a result, the focus shifts to lack of nutritional adequacy as a precondition for participation in labour market activities. Even if some succeed in participating, their wage earnings will not allow them to escape the PNT. Indeed, a mild labour market shock (associated with a crop shortfall) would worsen their plight, as the risk of loss of employment would be considerably higher. In particular, female workers are more prone to PNT than male workers, and there is persistent gender inequality in rural India. Breaking these traps should be a matter of urgent policy concern. We show that improving nutrient intakes can have significant effects on rural wages, and therefore, on the possibility of breaking the PNT as well as reducing poverty in rural India.

NOTES

1. In this chapter we use the terms efficiency wage hypothesis and PNT interchangeably. This is an adaptation of Jha *et al.* (2009a). The estimation procedure is informed by Dasgupta and Ray (1986, 1987) and Dasgupta (1993, 1997).
2. In an exception, Lakdawala *et al.* (2005) found that micronutrient deficiency needed to be considered in addition to calorie deficiency in the case of the U.S., and conjectured that this was probably also true of developing countries.
3. From a policy perspective, it is likely to be more useful to test for PNT for different nutrients separately. An aggregate of deprivation across various nutrients is essentially arbitrary and does not indicate, which is the most pressing deprivation.
4. For an algebraic exposition, see Dasgupta and Ray (1986, 1987) and Dasgupta (1997).
5. The prediction of inequality generalizes to informal markets, and non-market institutions (for example, the household). For an extension in which time and history result in horizontal inequity, see Dasgupta (1997, 2009).
6. In a meticulous review of empirical evidence on demand elasticities for calories and also the reverse impact of nutrition on productivity, Svedberg (2000) offers a different perspective. Noting data shortcomings and use of different econometric techniques, he argues that the diversity reflects the actual situation: there is no general systematic relationship between calorie intake (or body size) and income across households in different directions (p. 54).
7. Although more recent data are available in the India Human Development Survey, 2004–5, we have not been able to update this analysis because of

time and budgetary constraints. It is widely recognized that the quality of the NCAER data is superior to NSS (Smith *et al.* 2007: 12). Moreover, the NCAER collects both income and expenditure data while the NSS collects only expenditure data.

8. All are at 1994 prices.

9. Also see Chapter 4 for a brief exposition of the Heckman self-selection procedure. As the context matters, this may seem repetitive, but is meant to help the reader.

10. As Table 6.4 indicates, the null of no selection bias (as captured by the statistical significance of Mills' lambda) is rejected for: (i) male harvest wages carotene; (ii) male harvest wages iron; and (iii) male harvest wages riboflavin. The standard errors are corrected for selection bias.

11. To avoid cluttering the text with numbers, the details are omitted.

7 Child Undernutrition in India

Raghav Gaiha, Raghbendra Jha, and
Vani S. Kulkarni

In recent years, there has been a growing realization that poverty is multidimensional and money-metric indicators such as minimum income or expenditure cannot adequately capture all these dimensions. Attention has therefore shifted to other indicators such as health status, that relate more closely to basic capabilities of individuals. An important point is that the correspondence between basic capabilities (for example, to live a healthy and productive life) and level of income is not so strong (Sen 1985, 1999).[1] It is, therefore, not surprising that a wide range of indicators including income/expenditure, health, and education reflect a diverse pattern in India during the last two decades. In fact, as emphasized in a recent study, while most indicators have continued to improve during the 1990s, social progress has followed diverse patterns, ranging from accelerated progress in some fields to slowdown and even regression in others.[2]

Anthropometric measures of child malnutrition rely on height, weight, skin-fold thickness, and age. Following the Waterlow 3-tier classification, the most commonly used measures of anthropometric failure are stunting (low height-for-age), wasting (low weight-for-height), and underweight (low weight-for-age) (Behrman and Deolalikar 1988; Nandy *et al.* 2005). Stunting is an indicator of chronic undernutrition, attributable to prolonged food deprivation, and/or disease or illness;

wasting is an indicator of acute undernutrition, caused by more recent food deprivation or illness; underweight is a composite indicator of both acute and chronic undernutrition. Until recently, these indices were compared against international reference population indicators collected in the U.S. by the National Centre for Health Statistics (NCHS).[3] Children whose measurements fall below –2z scores of the reference population median are considered undernourished: stunted, wasted, or underweight. Those with measurements below –3z scores are considered severely undernourished.

An important feature of these indicators is the overlap between them: some children who are stunted will also have wasting and/or be underweight; some children who have wasting will also be stunted and/or be underweight. So there is a need for a more comprehensive measure of child undernutrition. Such a measure is proposed below, and measured with a recent household survey conducted jointly by University of Maryland and National Council of Applied Economic Research (NCAER), using the recent WHO norms (2006b).

In a not-so-recent study, Svedberg (2000) emphasized that the conventional indices of anthropometric failure are not sufficient for measuring the overall prevalence of child undernutrition. Since being underweight (having low weight-for-age) is a product of stunting and wasting and not their sum, it misses some children who are considered undernourished by the other indices, thus producing an underestimate. If children with wasting, stunting, or those who are underweight are all considered undernourished, a new aggregate indicator is needed that encompasses all undernourished children, be they wasted and/or stunted and/or underweight. This index is referred to as a Composite Index of Anthropometric Failure (CIAF).[4] The present chapter focuses on this measure.

This chapter reviews the extent and severity of different (but conventional) indices of child malnutrition in India. A distillation of evidence on the underlying factors helps understand better India's slow progress in reducing child malnutrition. Herein, a review of the CIAF among five-year-old children is carried out, based on a recent study by Nandy *et al.* (2005). It also describes the salient features of the household survey, *India Human Development Survey 2005* (IHDS). Our main results are discussed in three parts: (i) we examine the links between the CIAF and poverty, among others, using cross-tabulations;

(ii) we report our econometric results on the determinants of CIAF. A major point of departure from the extant literature is the focus on food prices as determinants of the CIAF, besides income, mother's education, home environment, and location; and (iii) we examine the association between the CIAF and infectious diseases. The chapter concludes with some observations from a broad policy perspective.

CHILD UNDERNUTRITION IN INDIA FROM A GLOBAL PERSPECTIVE

A grim picture of child undernutrition is painted in the recent *Save the Children Report* (hereafter referred to as *SCR* 2012).

> Every hour of every day, 300 children die because of malnutrition. It is an underlying cause of more than a third of children's deaths—2.6 million every year....
>
> Even for those children who survive, long-term malnutrition causes devastating and irreversible damage. Lack of nutritious food, coupled with infections and illness means their babies and brains do not develop properly. At least 170 million children are affected by stunting.
>
> This means that not only are they too short for their age, they are also likely to enrol at school later and to do less well academically. For example, iodine deficiency, a type of malnutrition caused by a lack of specific nutrients, affects one-third of school children in developing countries, and is associated with a loss of 10–15 IQ points. Childhood malnutrition can lessen productivity—stunted children are predicted to earn an average of 20 per cent less when they become adults.
>
> If current trends continue, the lives of more than 450 children globally will be affected by stunting in the next 15 years. (*SCR* 2012: vi)

Various assessments of progress in ameliorating child malnutrition point to a pitifully slow progress, but with regional and country variation. *SCR 2012*, for example, remains pessimistic about achieving the Millennium Development Goal (MDG) of halving the proportion of malnourished children by 2015, taking into account a combination of global trends—climate change, volatile food prices, economic uncertainty, and demographic shifts. Another recent study (Stevens *et al.* 2012) is also pessimistic, but draws attention to different regional and country prospects. Using data over the period 1985 to 2011, and a sophisticated model, its assessment is that children's anthropometric status improved in developing countries, but there were major differences across regions and countries in trends, and in present nutritional status.[5] The probability that the MDG target will be achieved by developing countries on the assumption that post-2000 trends continue is barely 0.05. Regionally, it varies from almost 0 in Sub-Saharan Africa to 1 in two Latin American and Caribbean regions. Specific countries with probabilities exceeding 0.80 include Chile, Brazil, Mexico, and China. Svedberg (2006), however, is more optimistic as his assessment is that the progress towards the MDG at the global level is on track due to the large decline in stunting in China. In India, by contrast, where no notable decline in child stunting took place over the 1990s, the rate of decline over the 2001–15 period must be very high for the MDG to be realized.[6]

India is one of a few countries with the worst levels of prevalence of low birth weight, underweight, and stunting among children in BRIC and SAARC countries (IAMR 2011). 43 per cent (38 per cent) of children under five are moderately underweight (stunted) in India, while the corresponding figures are 6 per cent (11 per cent) in China, 23 per cent (14 per cent) in Sri Lanka, 31 per cent (37 per cent) in Pakistan, 39 per cent (43 per cent) in Nepal, and 41 per cent (36 per cent) in Bangladesh in 2000–7, though these estimates have gradually declined in India in the past three decades (Deaton and Dréze 2009; Svedberg 2010). Using the first two rounds of National Family Health Survey (NFHS) data in 1992–3 and 1998–9, Tarozzi and Mahajan (2007) show that an overall nutritional status of children under three years improved during the 1990s, but they also observed rural-urban disparity (in favour of urban children), as well as gender disparity which aggravated (in favour of boys).

A recent important study but with limited coverage, HUNGaMA (2011), throws new light on the extent and severity of malnutrition among five-year-old children, based on conventional indicators.[7] The main findings are summarized below.

Stunting is far more pervasive (58.8 per cent) than underweight (42.3 per cent). Wasting is much lower (11 per cent). Undernutrition rates vary with age, rising most sharply for stunting up to the age of three years and then decline, rise moderately for underweight and decline for wasting. Female children lose out on the initial advantage in nutritional status, but this varies with the indicator. Lower nutritional outcomes are observed for children exposed to unhygienic living conditions and poor child-care practices, particularly breastfeeding in infancy. This is more so among low income households with mothers lacking education. There is a glaring contrast between the Focus Districts (FD) and the best districts (BD) in the same state, and a more glaring one relative to districts in the better performing states in some, but not all indicators. Somewhat surprisingly, village level infrastructure does not significantly influence variation in undernutrition. *Anganwadi* centres are widespread and well used, primarily for immunization and partly for food.

One of the major claims of this report is a sharp reduction in the prevalence of child malnutrition. It is asserted that in the 100 FD, the prevalence of child underweight decreased from 53 per cent in 2004 (District Level Household and Facility Survey–2) to 42 per cent (HUNGaMA 2011), a 20.3 per cent reduction over a seven-year period with an annual rate of reduction of 2.9 per cent. This may, however, be misleading as different anthropometric standards are used in the two surveys (Viswanathan 2012).[8]

A distillation of three contributions that throw light on determinants of child undernutrition, based on different data sets, is given below.

Gaiha and Kulkarni (2005) analysed the determinants of stunting, based on Human Development Survey data for 1994, collected by NCAER. Some of the main findings are summarized below:[9]

- Stunting as a manifestation of cumulative nutritional and health deprivation persists even among (relatively) affluent households in rural India. There is, of course, some overlap between stunting and income deprivation, but some other factors influence stunting independently of income. The evidence in fact confirms that income has a weaker role in reducing stunting than, say, easier access to drinking water, and sanitation and hygiene facilities.
- The number of stunted children is inversely associated with the proportion of children under 24 months. This suggests that the cumulative effect of periods of nutritional and health stress is greater as children get older.[10] However, the proportion of female children under five years has no effect on stunting. The number of stunted children is positively related to the number of children under 5 years in a household, mainly because of a birth order effect. In fact,

a more detailed analysis based on the NFHS for 1992–93 suggests a pattern of *selective* neglect by birth order and sex composition of children.[11] Boys and girls with surviving siblings of only the opposite sex are better-off than children with no surviving older siblings. Conversely, children with two or more surviving same sex siblings are worse-off in terms of severe stunting (Gaiha and Kulkarni 2005).

- Of particular importance is women's autonomy in fertility decisions and allocation of household resources. Early marriages result in frequent pregnancies, low birth weight babies, lesser attention to them, and greater stunting.
- Village and home infrastructure in terms of easy access to drinking water, and sanitation and hygiene facilities have a significant impact on stunting. Awareness building must be combined with mobilization of community resources to ensure that such improvements occur quickly and are sustainable (Ruel *et al.* 2013).
- Inter-village variation in prices of food items is considerable, as a result of remoteness of location, limited transport facilities, and local market imperfections (for example, commitment to sell milk at a low price to a few large buyers against advance payment who then sell it at considerably higher prices). So there is a strong case for strengthening road and transportation network, and for promoting more competitive local markets.

In brief, while income matters in reducing stunting, a more autonomous role for women, improvements in hygiene and sanitation facilities, and more competitive local markets for food items deserve higher priority.

Another study (Gaiha *et al.* 2011), based on state-level data constructed from the third round of NFHS (2005–6), yields interesting insights into prevalence of underweight among children under five.[12]

- Proportion of underweight children under five years varies inversely with living standards (monthly per capita expenditure) and female literacy rate (as a proxy for mother's education). The residuals of undernutrition (that is, the difference between actual and predicted values or 'excess' of undernutrition) diminish with media exposure (that is, newspaper circulation) but at a slower rate, as implied by the positive and significant coefficient of its square.[13] This implies that the greater the media exposure, the lower would be the gap between the actual and predicted proportions of underweight children. In other words, the lower would be the prospects of excess of underweight children. This evidence is suggestive of the role of the media in averting child undernutrition—even though it is not so visible.[14]

- Another interesting finding is that 'predicted' prevalence of underweight children is positively related to under 5 mortality. Our simulations show that if the proportion of underweight children falls by 10 per cent, the (mean) mortality rate falls by a little more than 10 per cent.

Among the most comprehensive studies is Imai *et al.* (2012), based on three rounds of the NFHS and two rounds of the NCAER data (*Human Development Survey* 1994, and *India Human Development Survey* 2004–5). Using state-of-art econometric models, it focuses on mother's bargaining power relative to father's on child malnutrition, measured in z scores of weight-for-height (wasting), height-for-age (stunting), and weight-for-age (underweight). Some of the important findings are summarized below.[15]

- More children under 5 years tend to result in worse nutritional outcomes for children. Boys under 3 are worse nourished than girls. A wealth index improves z scores and thus wealthier households have lower prevalence of child malnutrition. Women's bargaining index measured as a ratio of their schooling relative to father's positively and significantly influences z scores of weight-for-age (or underweight) as well as height-for-age (stunting)—at the low end of conditional distribution of z scores, implying improvements in these indicators. Children from SCs and STs tend to have lower z scores, implying worse child malnutrition.
- Access to health related facility, infrastructure, and environment are important factors in reducing the prevalence of child malnutrition. For example, wider access to a flush toilet is likely to improve nutritional status of children in terms of stunting and underweight. Easier access to drinking water reduces wasting. Access to radio and television reduces stunting and underweight.

- There is robust confirmation of many of the earlier results and new insights emerge into the favourable effects of women's empowerment on child malnutrition.

COMPOSITE INDEX OF ANTHROPOMETRIC FAILURE

Towards the objective of constructing the CIAF, Svedberg (2000) identifies six groups of undernourished children, as shown in Table 7.1. The sum of groups 2–7 constitutes a measure of total undernourished. Dividing this by the sum of groups 1–7 and multiplying by 100 gives the proportion of children undernourished. Following this procedure, an empirical analysis was conducted by Nandy *et al.* (2005), based on NFHS–2. The estimates of anthropometric failure were constructed for the age-group 0–3 years and are given in the last column of Table 7.1.[16]

45 per cent of children were stunted, 47 per cent were underweight, and 16 per cent were wasted. The CIAF was considerably higher (about 60 per cent) than any of these indicators.

Of the six sub-groups of undernourished children, those stunted and underweight accounted for well over one-fourth of the children, with all other sub-groups accounting for substantially lower shares. Those simultaneously wasted, stunted, and underweight accounted for about 7 per cent of the sample.

Their findings on negative health effects corroborate the usefulness of the disaggregated classification of undernourished children.[17] Those with multiple anthropometric failures (wasted and underweight, wasted, underweight and stunted, and stunted and underweight) were more likely to suffer from diarrhoea and acute respiratory infection (ARI) than those with only a single failure (wasted only, or stunted only). Those who were simultaneously wasted, stunted, and underweight were, in fact, the most likely to suffer from diarrhoea. Although analysis of risk of dying from these infectious diseases is rendered difficult by lack of anthropometric data on the dead and survivor bias, longitudinal data confirm that undernutrition (wasting and underweight) was twice as common among deceased children (Boerma *et al.* 1992).[18]

In sum, the disaggregation of undernourished children offers useful insights into risks of infectious diseases. These risks are aggravated for poor children given their limited access to health care.

TABLE 7.1 Classification of Undernourished Children (under 3 years)

Group	Description	Wasting	Stunting	Underweight	% Children
1.	**No Failure**: Children whose height and weight are above the age-specific norms (i.e., above −2 z scores) and do not suffer from any anthropometric failure	No	No	No	40.2
2.	**Wasting only**: Children with acceptable weight and height for their age but who have sub-normal weight for height	Yes	No	No	2.6
3.	**Wasting and underweight**: Children with above normal heights but whose weight for age and weight for height are too low.	Yes	No	Yes	6.1
4.	**Wasting, stunting, and underweight**: Children who suffer from anthropometric failure on all three measures.	Yes	Yes	Yes	7.2
5.	**Stunting and underweight**: Children with low weight-for-age but who have acceptable weight, both for their age and for their short height.	No	Yes	Yes	27.9
6.	**Stunting only**: Children with low height-for-age but who have acceptable weight, both for their age and for their short height.	No	Yes	No	10.1
7.	**Underweight only**: Children who are only underweight.	No	No	Yes	5.9
8.	**CIAF (=2+3+4+5+6+7) or =100−(1)**				**59.8**

Source: Svedberg (2000, pp. 194–6).

Note: The estimates of undernutrition were obtained from Nandy *et al.* (2005). Note that the combination of wasted and stunted is not physically possible since a child cannot simultaneously experience stunting and wasting, and not be underweight.

Our analysis is based on a nationwide household survey, *IHDS 2005*, conducted jointly by University of Maryland and NCAER. As salient features of this survey are described in Chapter 4, we have not repeated them here.

Two familiar problems with anthropometric data may be noted. One is the large number of children in the sample without anthropometric measurements, or those whose measurements are improbable (about 46 per cent).[19] So the small sample may be biased, but the nature and magnitude of the bias are uncertain.[20]

RESULTS BASED ON IHDS 2004–5

Let us first consider cross-tabulations of conventional indicators of anthropometric failure among five-year-old children. Note that these are obtained using the recent WHO (2006) norms.

Cross Tabulations of Anthropometric Failures

Prevalence rates of children being underweight (41 per cent) and stunted (36 per cent) are high—especially the former. Wasting is relatively low, but still afflicts about one-fifth of children under five years of age. What is also worrying is that nearly half of underweight and stunted children are severely so.

We then examine whether there is a large overlap between poverty and child undernutrition. Specifically, the question is whether undernutrition is largely a manifestation of poverty. Using the official poverty line, we construct cross-tabulations of different measures of child undernutrition and poverty status.[21] The contrast between poor and non-poor households is striking. Prevalence of underweight is markedly higher among poor children (47 per cent) than among the non-poor (39 per cent). Severely underweight children account for just under one-fourth of poor children as against under one-fifth of non-poor children. However, going by their shares in total underweight children, the non-poor underweight children accounted for just under two-thirds of the total. These findings imply that, while poor children are more likely to be underweight, the number of non-poor underweight children far exceeds that of the poor. Although income deprivation is closely related to the prevalence of underweight, other factors (for example, home environment, location, maternal care) are important too.[22]

As in the case of underweight, prevalence of stunting is much higher among poor children (41 per cent among the poor and 34 per cent among the non-poor), as also of severe stunting (22 per cent among the poor and 18 per cent among the non-poor). However, the number of non-poor stunted children far exceeds that of poor children, as also that of severely stunted children. The conclusion, therefore, is that factors associated with stunting are not confined to income deprivation—indeed, other factors (for example home environment, location, maternal care) matter as well.[23]

Prevalence rates of wasting do not vary much between the poor and non-poor children (about 22 per cent). Also, prevalence of severe wasting is nearly equal (about 9 per cent). However, the number of non-poor wasting children far exceeds that of the poor. These results also point to factors that go beyond income deprivation.

Our results point to more pervasive anthropometric failure in terms of the CIAF, relative to conventional indicators of being underweight, stunted, or wasted. The CIAF is about 59 per cent. Among the sub-categories, stunting and underweight, and stunting alone account for well over half of the CIAF. Children who fail in all three dimensions (simultaneously wasted, stunted, and underweight) account for a non-negligible share (13.5 per cent). The underweight alone account for the lowest share (about 6 per cent).

The contrast between the poor and non-poor children is striking (Table 7.2). The CIAF is considerably higher among poor children than among the non-poor. However, the number of poor children suffering from any of the anthropometric failures is considerably lower than that of non-poor. Among poor children, the proportion of both stunted and underweight children was highest, followed by that of stunted alone, and then wasted and underweight, and simultaneously wasted, stunted, and underweight. If we go by the shares of sub-groups of poor undernourished children in total of each, stunted and underweight children account for just under 39 per cent of the total, followed by the wasted, stunted, and underweight (under 38 per cent).

We now turn to anthropometric failure by location. The cross-tabulation of anthropometric failure by location (rural, metro, and non-metro urban areas) points to the following inferences.[24] The CIAF is highest in rural areas—over 60 per cent of under five-year-old children are afflicted in one way or another—followed by metros (over 54 per cent), and non-metro urban areas (under 53 per cent). These estimates imply that anthropometric failure affects not just rural areas, but also urban areas. However, more than three-fourths of the children suffering from diverse anthropometric failures lived in rural areas, and relatively small shares in non-metro urban areas (about 16.50 per cent) and metros (just under 6 per cent).

Turning to the sub-categories, the most pervasive or prevalent is stunting and underweight. A little over one-fifth of the rural children were afflicted by these failures, followed by lower shares in non-metro urban areas (under 15 per cent) and then metros (about 4.50 per cent). However, a vast majority of the total (under 81 per cent) were in rural areas.

The triple failure of stunting, wasting, and underweight is under 9 per cent in rural areas, and slightly lower in metros (over 6 per cent) and in non-metro urban areas (under 6 per cent). As in other cases, rural areas accounted for the largest share of the total (over 82 per cent).

In sum, the CIAF and its disaggregation into sub-categories of undernourished five-year-old children reveal a grimmer story of child undernutrition than conventional anthropometric indicators do. Not only is the prevalence of undernutrition in its diverse forms higher,

TABLE 7.2 Sub-Groups of Child Undernutrition and CIAF by Poverty Status in India in 2004–5

Groups	Share of Under 5 Children (%)	
	Poor	Non-Poor
1. No Failure	36.46 (28.82)	43.74 (71.18)
2. Wasting Only	6.26 (29.84)	7.15 (70.16)
3. Wasting and Underweight	9.80 (34.05)	9.22 (65.95)
4. Wasting, Stunting and Underweight	9.11 (37.62)	7.34 (62.38)
5. Stunting and Underweight	23.57 (38.92)	17.97 (61.08)
6. Stunting Only	11.04 (32.54)	11.11 (67.46)
7. Underweight Only	3.76 (34.44)	3.48 (65.56)
CIAF (=2+3+4+5+6+7)	63.54 (35.42)	56.26 (64.58)

Source: Authors' calculations based on IHDS, 2005.

Note: Figures within brackets are shares of total or each group.

but also simultaneous occurrence of anthropometric failures (for example, stunting and underweight, and stunting, wasting, and underweight) varies from moderate to high. Although poor children in general are more vulnerable to these failures, it is the non-poor or (relatively) affluent children who account for significantly larger shares of total undernourished children. Locationally, rural children are not just most prone to failures in any of the anthropometric dimensions and their simultaneous occurrence, but also account for the large majority of total undernourished children.

Determinants of Anthropometric Failures

As cross-tabulations do not simultaneously control for the effects of correlates other than those considered individually, we have carried out a regression analysis of the factors associated with the CIAF.

A regression model is specified, and estimated with individual and household data.[25] A general form of the regression model, as it applies to all n observations, is:

$$\mathbf{y} = \mathbf{X}\boldsymbol{\beta} + \boldsymbol{\varepsilon} \tag{1}$$

where $\mathbf{y}$ represents a column vector of all n observations on the dependent variable, the CIAF in each household, $\mathbf{X}$ is an n x K data matrix of K explanatory variables, and $\boldsymbol{\varepsilon}$ is a column vector of n disturbances. Given that the dependent variable is a composite household index, some important individual characteristics could not be considered, such as a child's age, gender, and birth order.

First, the regression is estimated using ordinary least squares (OLS). After checking for heteroscedasticity, a robust regression that adjusts the standard errors accordingly is estimated.

As the Breusch-Pagan test statistic ($\chi^2_1 = 21.27$) rejects homoscedasticity, our comments relate to robust regression results in Table 7.3. Let us first consider the regression coefficients.

Age of household head and the composite index are negatively related. That is, the higher the age, the lower was the index. There is no significant relationship between this index and caste, gender of the household head, and marital status of the household head (the spouses living together). However, the schooling years of the household head has

TABLE 7.3 Regression Analysis of Factors Associated with CIAF: Robust Regression

Explanatory Variables	Specification 1		Specification 2	
	Coefficient (t-value)	Elasticity	Coefficient (t-value)	Elasticity
Age: Household Head	−0.001*(−1.66)	−0.071	−0.001(−0.95)	−0.041
SC	0.018(0.79)	0.006	0.017(0.74)	0.006
ST	0.013(0.36)	0.002	0.009(0.24)	0.001
OBC	0.021(1.03)	0.012	0.018(0.92)	0.011
Gender: Household Head	0.016(0.28)	0.001	0.031(0.56)	0.002
Marital Status: Household Head	0.022(0.51)	0.033	0.020(0.46)	0.030
Years of Education: Household Head	−0.005**(−2.01)	−0.041		
Highest Years of Education: Female			−0.004*(−1.82)	−0.037
Highest Years of Education: Male			0.001(0.43)	0.012
Number of Children (0–5 years)	−0.045***(−3.34)	−0.099	−0.045***(−3.26)	−0.098
Household Kitchen with Vent	−0.062***(−2.94)	−0.037	−0.060***(−2.80)	−0.036
Piped water	0.033(1.30)	0.025	0.031(1.20)	0.023
Hand pump or tube-well	0.039(1.49)	0.024	0.038(1.44)	0.024
Rural areas	0.049*(1.85)	0.053	0.049*(1.85)	0.053
Urban metros	0.120***(3.32)	0.013	0.121***(3.35)	0.013
Log PCME	−0.113***(−3.50)	−0.184	−0.126***(−3.63)	−0.205
Log Price: rice	0.022(0.52)	0.035	0.022(0.51)	0.035
Log Price: wheat	−0.121***(−2.64)	−0.197	−0.113**(−2.46)	−0.184
Log Price: sugar	0.182*(1.82)	0.295	0.184*(1.84)	0.299

(continued)

TABLE 7.3 Continued

Explanatory Variables	Specification 1		Specification 2	
	Coefficient (t-value)	Elasticity	Coefficient (t-value)	Elasticity
Log Price: kerosene	−0.041(−0.86)	−0.067	−0.046(−0.94)	−0.074
Log Price: other cereals	−0.019(−0.91)	−0.032	−0.019(−0.87)	−0.030
Log Price: cereal-product	0.047(1.35)	0.076	0.048(1.39)	0.078
Log Price: pulses	−0.129★★★(−3.23)	−0.210	−0.128★★★(−3.18)	−0.208
Log Price: meat	−0.001(−0.05)	−0.002	−0.002(−0.08)	−0.004
Log Price: gur/sugar	−0.037(−1.47)	−0.060	−0.037(−1.45)	−0.060
Log Price: edible oil	−0.078(−0.82)	−0.127	−0.080(−0.84)	−0.131
Log Price: eggs	0.075★(1.70)	0.122	0.072^{w}(1.62)	0.116
Log Price: milk	0.054(0.93)	0.088	0.048(0.82)	0.078
Log Price: milk-product	−0.009(−0.71)	−0.015	−0.010(−0.75)	−0.016
Log Price: vegetables	0.045(1.50)	0.073	0.044(1.46)	0.071
Log Price: salt-spices	−0.056(−0.79)	−0.091	−0.053(−0.74)	−0.085
Log Price: tea-coffee-processed	−0.015(−0.35)	−0.024	−0.017(−0.39)	−0.027
Log Price: paan-tobacco	0.013 (1.56)	0.021	0.013 (1.54)	0.021
Log Price: fruits-nuts	0.011 (0.25)	0.018	0.029 (0.65)	0.047
Constant	1.670		1.689	
Number of observations	4603		4606	
F (32,4570)	7.34★★★		7.10★★★	

Source: Authors' calculations based on IHDS, 2005.

Note: ★★★, ★★, and ★ refer to significance at the 1 per cent, 5 per cent, and 10 per cent levels respectively; w denotes weak significance at > the 10 per cent level. All prices are at the PSU level.

a significant negative effect on the composite index of undernutrition of the children. This implies that the higher the educational attainment, the lower was the aggregate nutritional deprivation. Somewhat surprisingly, the larger the number of five-year-old children, the lower was the composite failure. We expected that the larger the number of children, the greater will be the competition for scarce food and medical care. Since the coefficient in question is negative, it implies the more significant effect of economies of scale in food expenditure. General hygiene in the kitchen—the presence of a vent—was negatively related to aggregate nutritional deprivation. Somewhat surprisingly, access to piped water, hand-pumps, or tube wells had no effect. Whether this effect is dampened by the fact that most households in urban areas have access to piped water needs further investigation. As expected, both rural areas and metros had higher aggregate anthropometric failures compared with non-metro urban areas. The higher the log of per capita expenditure, the lower was the composite failure.

There are significant price effects too.[26] As demonstrated in Chapter 3, price changes induce substitutions between different food commodities (including between different grades of, say, rice, vegetables), and thus in nutrient intakes. The present specification, however, does not allow us to ascertain the effects on nutrient intakes. So our comments are confined to just which price effects are significant. Note that these prices are in logs and were constructed at the PSU level (villages in rural areas).

Among cereals, the price of wheat has a significant negative effect on the composite index. This implies that higher wheat prices lower the composite index, as cheaper and more nourishing cereals (inferior cereals) are substituted.[27] A similar negative effect is associated with pulses, implying again substitutions of cheaper, protein-rich substitutes. By contrast, the higher the sugar and egg prices, the higher is the composite anthropometric failure, implying cheaper substitutes are less nourishing. Somewhat surprising is the absence of a positive effect of the price of milk.

As statistically significant effects of variables may not be necessarily large, we comment briefly on the (absolute) magnitudes of their elasticities. The elasticities (absolute) of CIAF with respect to quality of the kitchen, schooling years of household head, age of household head, and number of five-year-old children in the household are small. All of them have a negative sign. Location effects are positive and large, with that of rural areas considerably larger (more than four times) than that of metros (both relative to non-metro urban areas); income matters a great deal with higher incomes, reducing considerably the prevalence rate of aggregate nutritional deprivation.

Somewhat surprising is that none of the caste variables have a significant coefficient. In striking contrast, the elasticities of CIAF, with respect to prices of food commodities (sugar, pulses, and wheat) are larger than that of income. For instance, the elasticity is highest for sugar, followed by those of pulses, wheat, oil, and eggs. The price of vegetables, by contrast, has a (relatively) small, but weakly significant effect.

Similar results are obtained when household head's education is replaced by highest education of adult males and females (the latter as a proxy for mother's education). As shown in the last two columns of Table 7.3, only the education of adult female has a significant negative effect on the CIAF. The elasticity, however, is lower than expected. But the negative effect is consistent with a widely reported result that maternal education level is associated with lower child undernutrition. A familiar explanation is that better educated mothers ensure better medical care and healthier diets for their children. Indeed, it is arguable that women's empowerment has an important role in reducing child undernutrition (Gaiha and Kulkarni 2005; Imai *et al.* 2012).

In sum, household characteristics—specifically, mother's education, quality of kitchen, poverty, and location (whether in a rural area or in a metro)—are linked to aggregate anthropometric failure. Income matters a great deal in reducing CIAF. More important, however, are the effects of a few food prices. Although their influence through changes in nutrient intakes could not be identified, their reduced-form effects are strong.

Infectious Diseases and Anthropometric Failure

Svedberg (2000, 2007) and Nandy *et al.* (2005) sought to validate the disaggregated classification of undernutrition of children by linking it to susceptibility to infectious diseases such as diarrhoea, severe diarrhoea, and ARI. A result of particular significance is that children suffering from more than one anthropometric failure are more susceptible to these diseases than those suffering from no failure, or just one failure (with a few exceptions). Our analysis with the IHDS also focuses on these links, but the results are mixed, as shown below.

Except for wasted and underweight, and stunted only, in all other groups the prevalence of diarrhoea was higher than in the reference group of no failure. The highest prevalence rate was among those children who were simultaneously stunted and underweight, and those who were wasted, underweight, and stunted. That these differences are statistically significant is confirmed by the t-test.

In brief, there is support for the disaggregated classification of undernourished children for understanding better the prevalence of infectious diseases. Specifically, those with more than one failure were worse-off in this respect than children with no failure.

The differences in the prevalence of ARI are less striking. The highest prevalence occurs among stunted and underweight, followed by wasted and underweight children. Somewhat surprisingly, children with the triple failure of wasting, stunting, and underweight had a lower prevalence rate than that of no failure. However, only the difference between stunted and underweight, and no-failure children was statistically significant.

★★★

Some observations are made from a broad policy perspective. India is one of a few countries with the worst levels of low birth weight, stunting, and underweight among children in BRIC and SAARC countries. Despite rapid economic growth in the last two decades, the progress in reducing child undernutrition has been slow. Against this background, our analysis focused on the prevalence of CIAF among children under five years of age that refines the Waterlow 3-tier classification, using a nationwide household survey.

The CIAF and its disaggregation into sub-categories of undernourished five-year-old children reveal a grimmer story of child undernutrition than conventional anthropometric indicators do. Besides, simultaneous occurrence of anthropometric failures (stunting and underweight, and stunting, wasting, and underweight) is pervasive.

Our analysis of determinants of CIAF yields some new insights. Briefly, household characteristics—specifically, a (proxy for) mother's education, quality of kitchen, poverty, and location (whether in a rural area or in a metro)—are all linked to aggregate anthropometric failure. Income matters a great deal in reducing the CIAF. More important, however, are some food price effects, as they induce substitution between food commodities. Although their influence through changes in nutrient intakes could not be identified, their impacts are strong.

Investigation of the links between different anthropometric failures and prevalence of infectious diseases (diarrhoea and ARI) justifies the disaggregated classification of undernourished children used here. Specifically, those with more than one failure were worse-off in this respect than children with no failure.

There is a strong case for accelerating income growth together with food price stabilization in curbing child undernutrition. Female education has the desired effect, but it is less strong than expected. Indeed,

TABLE 7.4 Anthropometric Failure and Infectious Diseases

Anthropometric Group	Diarrhoea		t-value	Acute Respiratory Infection (ARI)		t-value
	% Share	Ratio		% Share	Ratio	
1. No Failure	26.61	1.0		47.49	1.0	
2. Wasting Only	29.57	1.11	−0.99	45.29	0.95	0.54
3. Wasting and Underweight	25.53	0.95	0.43	50.37	1.06	−0.86
4. Wasting, Stunting, and Underweight	31.96	1.20	−1.95*	44.74	0.94	0.77
5. Stunting and Underweight	32.82	1.23	−3.34**	53.97	1.14	−2.75**
6. Stunting Only	26.56	0.99	0.02	47.74	1.01	−0.08
7. Underweight Only	30.67	1.15	−1.11	46.83	0.99	0.14

Source: Authors' calculations based on IHDS, 2005.

Notes: Ratio represents proportions suffering from a disease in an undernourished group divided by the proportion of no failure. Accordingly, the t-test is a comparison of the differences in mean proportions of no failure group and of those suffering from a disease in each undernourished group.

* Denotes significance at the 5 per cent level; ** denote significance at the 1 per cent level.

higher female education relative to male education as a measure of women's empowerment has a favourable effect on child undernutrition. Improvement in the quality of home environment makes a difference too, but it is not conditional on income or wealth alone. Awareness of household hygiene and sanitation needs inculcation—especially in rural areas. Rural-urban disparity, reflecting largely disparity in access to infrastructure and medical services, continues to dampen progress in reducing child undernutrition.

From this perspective, a priority is to strengthen the Integrated Child Development Services (ICDS) and a better synchronization with the Rural Health Mission (RHM). A finding of considerable policy significance from the experience of several developing countries—including India—is that combined early child development and nutrition interventions have additive or synergistic effects on child development and could lead to substantial gains in cost, efficiency, and effectiveness (Ruel *et al.* 2013).

Finally, as it is a form of 'hidden' hunger, the potential for reduction through greater media exposure should not be overlooked.

ANNEXURE

TABLE 7A.1 Definitions of Variables Used in the Analysis

Variable	Definition
Dependent variable	
CIAF	Composite Index of Anthropometric Failure
Explanatory variables	
Age: Household Head	Age (in years)
SC	=1 if social group is SC; 0 otherwise
ST	=1 if social group is ST; 0 otherwise
OBC	=1 if social group is OBC; 0 otherwise
Others (reference)	Omitted group
Gender: Household Head	=1 if household head is female; 0 if male
Marital Status: Household Head	=1 if household head is married; 0 otherwise
Highest Years of Education: Adult Female	Highest years completed in education by a female household member

(continued)

TABLE 7A.1 Continued

Variable	Definition
Highest Years of Education: Adult Male	Highest years completed in education by a male household member
Household Kitchen with Vent	=1 if kitchen has vent; 0 otherwise
Piped water	=1 if access to piped water; 0 otherwise
Hand pump or tube-well	=1 if household has hand pump or tube-well; 0 otherwise
Rural areas	=1 if Rural, 0 otherwise
Urban metros	=1 if Metro, 0 otherwise
Non-metro urban (reference)	=1 if Non-metro urban, 0 otherwise
Marital Status Household Head: Married	=1 if household head is married; 0 otherwise
Log PCME (IV)	Log of per capita monthly expenditure (predicted-)
Log Price: rice[1]	Log Price of rice
Log Price: wheat	Log Price of wheat
Log Price: sugar	Log Price of sugar
Log Price: kerosene	Log Price of kerosene
Log Price: other-cereals	Log Price of other-cereals
Log Price: cereal-product	Log Price of cereal-product
Log Price: pulses	Log Price of pulses
Log Price: meat	Log Price of meat
Log Price: *gur*	Log Price of *gur*
Log Price: edible oil	Log Price of edible oil
Log Price: eggs	Log Price of eggs
Log Price: milk	Log Price of milk
Log Price: milk-product	Log Price of milk-product
Log Price: vegetables	Log Price of vegetables
Log Price: salt-spices	Log Price of salt-spices
Log Price: tea-coffee-processed	Log Price of tea-coffee-processed
Log Price: *paan*-tobacco	Log Price of *paan*-tobacco
Log Price: fruits-nuts	Log Price of fruits-nuts

Source: IHDS, 2005.

Note: All prices are at the PSU level.

NOTES

1. There is a great deal of variability between low capabilities, such as undernourishment, and low incomes, and this relationship is conditional, differing by community, families, and individuals. More specifically, the contribution of income or expenditure to explaining health outcomes is limited. Sahn and Stifel (2002), for example, report that the correlation coefficient between a wealth index derived using factor analysis and a health indicator ranges from 0.081 to 0.243 in a sample of 10 countries.

2. For details, see Deaton and Drèze (2009). See also a meticulous analysis by Svedberg (2010) to reconcile different estimates of child malnutrition based on NHFS and NNMB.

3. These norms are now replaced by substantially revised ones prepared by WHO (2006).

4. In a more recent contribution, Nandy *et al.* (2005) further illustrate the relevance of this composite index using estimates of separate anthropometric failure and the composite index for a few countries. Without rejecting the use of separate indicators, he argues that the CIAF is also justified because it is important to know the overall scale of the problem, so that sufficient resources are allocated to it. A few illustrations are useful. The CIAF as an overall measure of undernutrition shows India and Ethiopia had the highest prevalence rates. The difference between this index and underweight in the countries analysed was more than ten percentage points. Hence underweight as an indicator clearly misses numbers of undernourished children. Moreover, while underweight in India and Peru show fall in relative terms of around 11 per cent, the CIAF shows limited progress, with relative fall of only 6 and 4 per cent, respectively. This raises serious doubts about using underweight as an indicator for progress towards the first MDG.

5. A Bayesian hierarchical mixture model is used to analyse anthropometric distributions. For details, see Stevens *et al.* (2012).

6. This assessment is refuted by Stevens *et al.* (2012) on the grounds that it did not carry out a systematic analysis of global trends and was confined to a small number of countries selected based on their total population, even though the global trend is affected most by countries with the largest number of underweight children. But it cannot be ruled out that Svedberg may have reached different conclusions with access to more recent data on child undernutrition.

7. The HUNGaMA survey, initiated by the Citizens' Alliance against Malnutrition, and coordinated by the Naandi Foundation, Hyderabad, was conducted in 3,360 villages across nine states between October 2010 and February 2011. The 100 focus districts (FD) were identified on the basis of low ranks in a child development district index constructed for UNICEF in

India in 2009. These districts are in Bihar, Jharkhand, Madhya Pradesh, Orissa, Rajasthan, and Uttar Pradesh. Along with these districts, the survey also covered the best performing districts in each of these states and two districts each in Himachal Pradesh, Kerala, and Tamil Nadu for comparison. At the individual level, the survey measured height, weight, and mid upper-arm circumference (MUAC) of 1.09 lakh children below the age of five years, constituting about 20 per cent of the children in this age group in 2011. At the household level, data were gathered on child-care practices by 74,000 mothers. At the village level, data were collected on the services offered by *Anganwadis*. For further details, see the HUNGaMA report and, for a critique, Viswanathan (2012).

8. Besides, the regression analysis conducted by Banerjee and Zucker (2011) leaves much to be desired; specifically, (i) subsets of explanatory variables (for example, income and infrastructure) are used separately, raising doubts about the robustness of the coefficient estimates; (ii) food prices as explanatory variables are omitted, despite evidence to the contrary; and (iii) districts are not weighted by their populations.

9. This analysis is based on a 'Poisson' regression model.

10. Sahn and Stifel (2002) present evidence on catch-up growth after the weaning age.

11. Kulkarni *et al.* (2013) provides a review of more recent evidence reflected in number of missing girls.

12. The analysis is based on robust regression analysis.

13. Constrained by the data, we were unable to examine whether 'local' newspapers are more effective than national newspapers in English.

14. See, for example, Kapoor (2009) on the hidden hunger of children in India. She observes '... people respond immediately when they read about starvation deaths during famines and disasters. But it is less easy to evoke sympathy and support when the plight of the victims does not hit you squarely in the face. 90 per cent of malnutrition cases in India are of the chronically undernourished, where there are not necessarily obvious outward symptoms. Nevertheless this malnutrition doubles our infant mortality rate, making the child twice as susceptible to disease because of lowered immunity'.

15. We do not report differences in a few results depending on the econometric technique and anthropometric indicator used. Details are available in Imai *et al.* (2012).

16. The reference population is the NCHS.

17. These results were obtained from a binary logistic regression of diarrhoea, severe diarrhoea, and ARI on anthropometric failures. It is not clear whether any allowance was made for the endogeneity of anthropometric failures.

18. Boerma *et al.* (1992) and Svedberg (2000) also contain clear exposition of survivor bias.

19. In a total sample of 24,314 children in the age-group of 0–5 years, barely 13,524 had anthropometric measurements.
20. Whether these problems result in underestimation of undernutrition—as conjectured by Nandy *et al.* (2005)—seems plausible, but is subject to validation.
21. The average poverty line is Rs 356 per person per month in rural areas and Rs 538 in urban areas (Desai *et al.* 2010).
22. Details available on request.
23. Details available on request.
24. Details available on request.
25. Following the classification into mutually exclusive seven categories of single or multiple anthropometric failures, each child under five years in a household is classified into one of the categories. There is no question of the CIAF taking the value 0 since the sample is confined to children with anthropometric data. Suppose there is just one child (households with no children are excluded) under five years in a household, the CIAF will take the value 1 if there is no anthropometric failure, and he/she will be assigned to the category of no failure. Suppose there are two children with one stunted, the CIAF for category 6 will be 0.50 or 50 per cent. An important point here is that proportions of children will be assigned to different categories depending on the nature of anthropometric failure. So there will be several values of the CIAF and these are aggregated (each being a proportion of number of children under five years) to obtain a household measure of CIAF (or the total burden of undernutrition).
26. For an earlier corroboration of food price effects in explaining anthropometric failure, see Gaiha and Kulkarni (2005).
27. More expensive grades of weight were consumed, perhaps because of taste and flavour considerations.

8 Affluence, Obesity, and Non-communicable Diseases in India

Raghav Gaiha, Raghbendra Jha, and Vani S. Kulkarni

The dietary transition involves not just a more varied and nutritionally balanced diet and higher levels of food hygiene, but also consumption of energy-dense foods that are linked to a higher prevalence of diet-related non-communicable diseases (NCDs). Although India lags behind other developing countries in the epidemiological transition—decline in infectious disease mortality compensated for increasingly by higher mortality from chronic degenerative NCDs—there is some evidence of this transition taking place.[1]

A recent World Bank study (2011) throws valuable light on the shifting disease burden in South Asia, risk factors associated with both NCDs and communicable diseases, costs and projections, and policies to avert deaths.

Ageing is increasing rapidly, but often without the social changes such as improved living conditions, better nutrition, and better access to health services that accompanied ageing in most developed countries much earlier.[2] Ageing alone is likely to increase NCDs as they are more common with increasing age.

Low birth weight is an important risk factor for NCDs. The foetal origins hypothesis of adult disease postulates that foetal undernutrition, reflected by low birth weight, is linked to susceptibility to ischemic heart disease and other chronic NCDs later in life. Foetal nutritional deprivation, followed by later excesses, lead to obesity and vulnerability to disease. Indian infants, for example, with poorly nourished mothers are born with weight deficits, but in relative terms, the deficits in lean mass are greater than those in adiposity. In later life, when high-energy and high-fat diets are consumed, the previously 'thin fat' babies also have greater central adiposity and vulnerability to disease (Popkin *et al.* 2012).[3]

Over half the disease burden (55 per cent including injuries) is now attributable to NCDs, a larger share than communicable diseases and maternal and child health (MCH) issues. Ischemic heart disease is the leading cause of both deaths and forgone disability adjusted life years (DALYs) in working age adults (15–69 years).[4] By contrast, communicable diseases (tuberculosis, respiratory infections, and water and vector-borne disease) are still prominent in the total population, reflecting a 'double disease burden'.

Chronic NCDs require treatment over a much longer period than acute communicable diseases. Given existing health financing patterns in many low and middle-income countries (the poorer a country is, the more regressive the health care financing system is, and the higher the fraction of costs borne by the patients themselves through out-of-pocket expenses), the costs associated with NCDs are likely to be a greater burden on those least likely to afford them (World Bank 2011).

Estimates of costs cannot be taken at face value except as illustrative. Projections suggest that, over the ten years from 2005, deaths from heart disease, stroke, and diabetes would lower GDP in India and Pakistan by 1 per cent from what it would have been without this burden. At the microeconomic level, if those affected are the main earners or those rearing children, NCD-related short-or long-term disability, or premature death, can cause drastic cuts in food and education expenditure and liquidation of assets (World Bank 2011).

A selective summary of India's key statistics is given below.[5]

The demographic transition is likely to advance in the future. The proportion of sixty-five years and older will rise from 4.4 per cent to 7.6 per cent in 2025.

In 2004, NCDs accounted for 62 per cent of the total burden of forgone DALYs, with the remainder from communicable diseases and

MCH issues. Of the total DALY burden, cardiovascular disease (CVD) accounts for 12.7 per cent; mental health for 11.6 per cent; cancer for 3.5 per cent; respiratory diseases for 4.6 per cent; diabetes for 1.1 per cent; and injuries for 12.5 per cent.

By 2030, CVD is expected to be the main cause of death (36 per cent). It occurs at an earlier age (compared to the rest of the world), has higher case fatality rates, and disease onset at lower risk factor thresholds, particularly for the overweight and obese.

Diabetes prevalence has increased in both rural and urban areas. The range for urban populations is 5–15 per cent, for semi-urban populations is 4–6 per cent, and for rural populations it is 2.5 per cent. Diabetes is increasing among the poor.

Hypertension affects 25 per cent of the urban and 10 per cent of the rural population.

Over 70 per cent of cancer cases are diagnosed during the advanced stages of the disease, resulting in poor survival and high mortality rates.

In a comprehensive study, Mahal *et al.* (2009) demonstrate that NCDs constitute a major economic burden in India. They report high levels of out-of-pocket spending by households with members suffering from NCDs, the limited levels of insurance coverage (including subsidized public services), and the income losses that befall affected households. Associated with these costs are risks of catastrophic spending and impoverishment, and, of course, macro impacts.[6]

NCDs share of total out-of-pocket health expenditures during 1995–2004 rose from 31.6 per cent to 47.3 per cent, pointing to a growing financial burden on households of NCDs. About 40 per cent of household expenditures for treating NCDs were financed by household borrowing and sales of assets. The odds of incurring catastrophic hospitalization expenditures were nearly 160 per cent higher with cancer than with a communicable disease. The odds of catastrophic hospital expenditures due to CVD were 30 per cent greater than for a communicable disease. Duration of illness, measured as days when people could not work, was in the range of 50–70 days for some NCDs, greater than that from other conditions.

The present chapter examines the prevalence of NCDs, and seeks to throw new light on the underlying factors, including socio-economic, demographic, and locational characteristics of households. Of particular importance are the links between growing affluence and NCDs.

A policy imperative is to address the 'double burden' of disease, but, more importantly, to avert the spectre of growing disabilities and deaths due to NCDs.

In the next section, we describe the salient features of the household survey on which this analysis is based, followed with a review of the prevalence rates of some NCDs (heart disease, diabetes, cancer) and their socio-economic correlates. Some of the key inter-relationships include demographic aspects of those suffering from such diseases (gender, age group), BMI as a measure of overweight and obesity, their standard of living (or relative affluence), caste affiliation, location (whether prevalence rates vary between rural and urban areas, as also between urban areas and urban slums), and lifestyle changes (whether eating out is associated with higher prevalence rates of some of these diseases). Subsequently, we analyse the factors underlying (average) incidence of NCDs and a related, but different variant in a household, followed by concluding observations from a broad policy perspective.

DATA

Our analysis is based on a nationwide household survey, *India Human Development Survey* (IHDS) 2005, conducted jointly by University of Maryland and National Council of Applied Economic Research (NCAER). IHDS covers over 41,000 households residing in rural and urban areas, selected from thirty-three states.[7] The sample comprises 384 districts out of a total of 593 identified in the 2001 population census. Villages and urban blocks constitute the primary sampling unit from which the households were selected.

As incidence of NCDs is self-reported, it has familiar limitations. The main problem is that we only observe the response to the statement, and the consequent bias.[8]

More details of the survey are given in Chapter 4.

CORRELATES OF NCDs

A broad brush treatment of the prevalence of NCDs and their correlates is given below.

As the classification into different NCDs (high blood pressure, heart disease, and diabetes) is not mutually exclusive, let us first consider the cases that overlap. As noted earlier, the analysis is confined to those above twenty-two years of age.[9] The overlap between high blood pressure and heart disease was about 21 per cent. The overlap between high blood pressure and diabetes was even higher (about 33 per cent). However, the overlap between heart disease and diabetes was somewhat low (about 7 per cent). Whatever the plausibility of these estimates, the importance of competing medical risks in classifying individuals, as well as in designing health policies, is reinforced (Mahal *et al.* 2009).

Demographic Aspects

Our review is confined to whether prevalence rates of different NCDs vary by gender and age group. To help assess relative magnitudes, shares of sub-samples by gender and age group are given. About 45 per cent were male and the remaining (about 55 per cent) were female. About 39 per cent were in the age group 23–45 years, and about 60 per cent in the older age group >45 years.

About 26 per cent of the sample individuals suffered from high blood pressure. Of these, a large majority (over 60 per cent) were females. Most (over 74 per cent) were also in the older age-group above forty-five years.

The prevalence rate of heart disease (over 9 per cent) was considerably lower, relative to high blood pressure. Of these, the majority (over 55 per cent) were females. As in the case of high blood pressure, the majority of those suffering from heart disease were in the older age-group, above forty-five years (66 per cent).

Those suffering from diabetes were just under 16 per cent of the sample. Among them, the majority (about 56 per cent) were male. As in the case of high blood pressure and heart disease, the majority of diabetics were in the older age-group, above forty-five years (78 per cent).

The prevalence of cancer (about 1.25 per cent) was relatively low. The majority of those reported to be suffering from it (about 58 per cent) were male. Most were also in the older age group above forty-five years (69 per cent).

Affluence and NCDs

As some of the NCDs (for example, heart disease) are closely associated with dietary transition, we examine below the links between these diseases and overweight/obesity.[10] A diagrammatic representation of

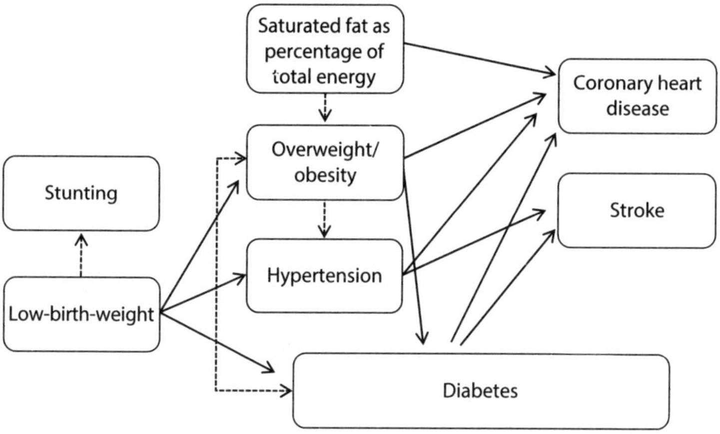

FIGURE 8.1 Relative Risks for Coronary Heart Disease, Stroke, and Diabetes
Source: Adapted from Popkin *et al.* (2001).

risk of diet-related factors associated with selected NCDs is given in Figure 8.1.[11]

For our descriptive analysis we use the following indicators of standard of living: (i) poverty status;[12] (ii) monthly per capita expenditure (MPCE)—we classify individuals as earning/spending less than Rs 300 per capita per month, between Rs 300 and Rs 500 per capita per month, between Rs 500 and Rs 1000 per capita per month, and more than Rs 1000 per capita per month; (iii) location—individuals are classified as living in rural, urban, and urban slums, with those living in rural areas and urban slums as generally worse-off than those living in urban areas; and (iv) caste—we classify individuals into Scheduled Castes (SCs), Scheduled Tribes (STs), Other Backward Castes (OBCs), and 'others'. The STs are typically the most poverty prone, followed by the SCs, and then the OBCs (Desai *et al.* 2010).

Given the poverty cut-off points, a small fraction of individuals was poor (just under 14 per cent). About 5 per cent of the individuals had MPCE of <Rs 300, about 19 per cent between Rs 300–500, about 41 per cent between Rs 500–1000, and about 35 per cent >Rs 1000. The sample individuals seem much better-off than nationally representative samples (the NSS) show, presumably because of the age cut-off and reporting bias. The majority lived in rural areas (under 70 per cent), a little under 30 per cent in urban areas, and a tiny fraction in urban slums (1.38 per cent). About 19 per cent were SCs, a little over 4 per cent were STs, a little over 37 per cent were OBCs, and over 39 per cent were 'others'.

The key findings based on these correlates of NCDs are discussed here.[13]

HIGH BLOOD PRESSURE

A vast majority of those reported to be suffering from high blood pressure (over 90 per cent) were non-poor. Also, among the non-poor, well over a quarter suffered from high blood pressure, while among the poor just one-fifth did. About 85 per cent of those suffering from high blood pressure were in the upper tail of the expenditure distribution (>Rs 500 per capita per month), while just over 2 per cent were in the lower tail (<Rs 300 per capita per month). What is also striking is that as the expenditure interval rises, the proportion suffering from high blood pressure also rises. The largest proportion of those suffering from high blood pressure (about 39 per cent) was in urban areas followed by those in urban slums (well over 35 per cent). A large proportion of those suffering from high blood pressure was among 'others' (49 per cent), followed by OBCs (34 per cent), and then the SCs (15 per cent) and STs (2 per cent). If 'others' are least prone to poverty and generally the most affluent, there is further support for a strong link between (relative) affluence and this condition. This is reinforced by the fact that nearly one-third of 'others' reported to be affected by this condition.

HEART DISEASE

A vast majority of those reported to be suffering from heart disease (over 90 per cent) were non-poor. Using the more detailed expenditure classification, we find that a large proportion of those suffering from heart disease (about 49 per cent) were in the upper tail of the income distribution (>Rs 1000 per capita per month) while barely 2 per cent were in the lower tail (<Rs 300 per capita per month). Also, the proportion suffering from this condition rises with the expenditure interval. The largest concentration of those suffering from

heart disease was in rural areas (57 per cent), followed by urban areas (41 per cent). The cross-classification of those suffering from heart disease by caste points to the most affluent group of 'others', accounting for the majority of those affected by this condition (over 52 per cent), while the most disadvantaged (the STs) were barely 1.50 per cent.

DIABETES

As in other NCDs, a vast majority of diabetics (about 93 per cent) were non-poor. Also, the proportion of the non-poor reporting this condition was twice as high as among the poor. In the more detailed expenditure classification, over 48 per cent of the diabetics were in the highest expenditure interval (>Rs 1000 per capita per month), while just under 2 per cent were in the lowest interval (<Rs 300 per capita per month). Also, the proportion of those reporting this condition in the highest expenditure interval was nearly five times that in the lowest interval. Diabetes is widely prevalent in rural areas (over 54 per cent), followed closely by urban areas (about 45 per cent).[14] However, among those in urban areas, about a quarter reported this condition, more than twice as high as in rural areas. As in other NCDs, the highest proportion of those suffering from diabetes were 'others' (over 47 per cent), followed by OBCs (about 38 per cent). Also, among 'others', the proportion of diabetics was highest (about 19 per cent) as compared with barely 3.60 per cent among STs.

CANCER

The vast majority of cancer cases (over 83 per cent) were reported among the non-poor. However, there was little difference in the proportions of the non-poor and poor, reporting this condition. Over 37 per cent of cancer cases were in the highest expenditure interval (>Rs 1000 per capita per month), followed by about 31 per cent in the next lower interval (Rs 500–1000 per capita per month), as compared with barely 4 per cent in the lowest expenditure interval (<Rs 300 per capita per month). The proportions of reported cancer cases among various expenditure groups, however, varied little. Just under three quarters of the cancer cases were in rural areas, followed by a little over a quarter in urban areas. Going by caste affiliation, about 43 per cent of cancer

cases were OBCs and over 37 per cent were 'others', as compared with barely 0.21 per cent among the STs—the most disadvantaged group.

In sum, there is ample evidence of strong links between NCDs and (relative) affluence. Besides, in some cases (for example, heart disease, diabetes, and cancer), the prevalence rates are high in rural areas. Since our results are based on cross-tabulations, the effects of other variables are not taken into account. We look at these links in more detail later, focusing on marginal effects of various household characteristics (socio-economic, demographic, and location). This allows us to isolate the effect of each characteristic controlling for the effects of others.

Obesity and NCDs

A feature of many low and middle-income countries is persistence of underweight, stunting and micronutrient deficiencies with increasing rates of obesity. This 'dual' burden of undernutrition and obesity exists not just within countries and communities, but also within the same household, and even in some individuals who may have excess adiposity along with micronutrient deficiencies, such as iron deficiency, anaemia, or stunting and overweight. Dual burden households are more common in countries undergoing nutrition transition (Popkin *et al.* 2012).

The emergence of this double burden is symptomatic of the nutrition transition underway in developing countries as a result of their growing prosperity and urbanization. Diets are shifting from traditional foods towards low-cost, energy-dense foods, high in salts, fats, and sugars. Physical activity patterns have become less strenuous and more sedentary.

The excess energy from these foods may affect children and adults within the same household differently. Children may use up the excess energy and still remain underweight, while adults are more likely to gain weight. Intra-household food allocation biases between adults and children on the one hand, and between male and female on the other, compound these effects.

Let us now consider the subset of households that contain both underweight children (under-five years) and obese adults. Although their share was low—about 3.30 per cent in the aggregate sample—it varied slightly between the poor and non-poor (2.35 per cent and 3.75 per cent, respectively). In a more disaggregated MPCE classification, there was, however, a clear progression, with the obesity rate rising from 2.85 per cent to 6.50 per cent. In the urban areas and urban slums, the rate (about 4.86 per cent) was almost twice as high as in the rural areas (2.75 per cent).[15]

First, let us consider how prevalent obesity is and whether it is linked to affluence. Note that the data used for constructing the body mass index (BMI) were collected for a relatively small sample, and selectively for a few adults in a household.[16] Following WHO norms, those with BMIs between 25–30 are classified as overweight, and those exceeding 30 are classified as obese.[17]

Given selective reporting of BMI, the estimates of normal, overweight, and obese must be interpreted with caution. Over 12 per cent of the sample individuals above twenty-two years were overweight, and over 3 per cent were obese. Under 50 per cent of the overweight and over 58 per cent of the obese were in urban areas. In contrast, the share of overweight was larger in rural areas (about 51 per cent) and that of obese was considerably lower (over 38 per cent). Vast majorities of both overweight and obese were non-poor (88 per cent and 91 per cent, respectively).

Let us now examine the links between obesity and NCDs. While the share of overweight among those suffering from high blood pressure is high (over 34 per cent), that of obese is low (about 12 per cent). However, the proportion reporting this condition was highest for the obese (about 43 per cent), followed by the overweight (about 37 per cent). Over 59 per cent of those reporting heart disease had BMI in the (normal) range of 18–25, over 20 per cent were overweight, and barely over 8 per cent were obese. However, the proportion reporting this condition was highest for the obese (over 13 per cent). A strong link between overweight or obesity and diabetes is not discernible, as the largest proportion of diabetics is in the normal range of BMI (18–25). However, of the obese, nearly a quarter reported this condition—by far the highest proportion of different ranges of BMI. As cancer in general is unlikely to be associated with being overweight or obese, any further comment is unnecessary.

We also investigated the link between eating out, and overweight and obesity. The main finding is that in the highest expenditure interval for eating out (Rs 500 per month), the proportion of overweight was over 22 per cent as against under 12 per cent among those who did not eat out at all. Also, the proportion of obese in this expenditure interval (over 6 per cent) was more than twice that in the households that did not eat out.

In sum, while being overweight or obese enhances the risk of NCDs, further investigation is necessary to isolate the effects of the former.[18]

DETERMINANTS OF NCDs

Methodology

As the cross-classifications cannot isolate the causal/associational relationships, we use two econometric specifications for isolating the effects of BMI, socio-demographic household characteristics, and location on the prevalence of NCDs. In the first specification, our dependent variable is average incidence of NCDs (that is, number of adult household members suffering from high blood pressure, or heart disease, or diabetes, or cancer per household size). In a variant, taking account of the fact that there are overlaps between various diseases (for example, between high blood pressure and heart disease, between diabetes and heart disease), and some adults report suffering from more than one ailment, we add up the number of ailments reported by household members and divide it by household size. As these averages cluster around zero or small values, a tobit specification is employed.[19]

Algebraically, the tobit model expresses the observed response, y, in terms of an underlying latent variable:

$$y^{\star} = \beta_0 + \boldsymbol{x\beta} + \mu, \quad \mu \,|\, \mathbf{x} \sim \text{Normal}\left(0, \sigma^2\right) \tag{1}$$

$$\text{y} = \max\left(0, \text{y}^{\star}\right) \tag{2}$$

The latent variable $y^{\star}$ satisfies the classical linear model assumptions; in particular, it has a normal homoscedastic distribution with a linear conditional mean. Equation (2) implies that the observed variable y equals $y^{\star}$ when $y^{\star} \geq 0$, but $y = 0$ when $y^{\star} < 0$. Since $y^{\star}$ is normally distributed, y has a continuous distribution over strictly positive values (Wooldridge 2006).

The unit of analysis is household. A selection of the results is discussed below.

Ageing, Affluence, Obesity and Incidence of NCDs

The analyses are premised on a health production function.[20] In the first specification of the average incidence of NCDs, the right side or explanatory variables include whether any adult is overweight or obese, gender of household head, age and age squared of household head, highest educational attainments of adult males and females, log of per capita expenditure, and caste affiliation (whether OBC, SC, or ST relative to 'others').

RURAL

The results are given in Table 8.1. We will first comment on the coefficients, and then on the elasticities.[21]

Overweight and obese adults are positively related to the prevalence of NCDs; age has a positive effect, but it diminishes with advancing age; education of adult females is positively related while that of adult males is negatively related to the prevalence of NCDs;[22] per capita expenditure has a positive effect; and SCs have higher prevalence, while STs have lower prevalence relative to 'others'.

If educated adult females (likely to be spouses) are more likely to have a say in cooking, it is plausible that they are likely to cook healthier diets (Gaiha *et al.* 2009). But a trade-off cannot be ruled out between outside employment and household chores, and a likely neglect of the latter.

Going by the absolute elasticities, the highest is with respect to age net of that of its square, confirming the important role of ageing in explaining the burden of NCDs. The next highest elasticity is with respect to per capita expenditure.[23] Education of both female and male adults have small elasticities. Somewhat surprising is the even smaller elasticity with respect to overweight/obese adults. Lowest elasticities are associated with SC and ST households—especially the latter.

TABLE 8.1 Tobit Analysis of Factors Associated with Average Incidence of NCDs—Rural India (2004–5)

Dependent Variable: Number of Household Members suffering divided by the household size	No. of observations = 3927 LR Chi^2 (10) = 365.34 Prob>Chi2 = 0.0000					
	Coefficient			Elasticity		
Obesity Dummy (=0 if BMI of any member is less than 25, else = 1)	0.109	(7.28)	***	0.025	(7.32)	***
Female headed household	−0.037	(−1.2)	**	−0.002	(−1.2)	**
Age of household head	0.014	(4.43)	***	1.002	(4.44)	***
Age of household head – squared	0.000	(−4.26)	***	−0.466	(−4.26)	***
Highest education level of female adults	0.008	(4.63)	***	0.046	(4.66)	***
Highest education level of male adults	−0.005	(−3.02)	***	−0.048	(−3.01)	***
Log of monthly per capita expenditure	0.190	(8.84)	***	0.277	(11.58)	***
Caste Dummy (SC)	0.038	(2.33)	**	0.014	(2.34)	**
Caste Dummy (ST)	−0.068	(−1.9)	**	−0.005	(−1.91)	**
Caste Dummy (OBC)	0.010	(0.71)	**	0.006	(0.71)	**
Constant	−1.697	(−11.34)				

Source: Authors' calculations based on IHDS, 2005.

Notes: Reference category for caste dummies: Others; ***, **, * denote significant at 1 per cent, 5 per cent, and 10 per cent, respectively.

Number of household members suffering from either high blood pressure, heart disease, diabetes, or cancer divided by household size.

URBAN

Some of the key results in the rural sample are reproduced in the urban sample, but the magnitudes differ, as given in Table 8.2. Overweight/obese adults are linked positively to the prevalence of NCDs; age has a positive effect, but it weakens with advancing age; per capita expenditure has a positive effect on the prevalence of NCDs. Neither education of adult females and males, nor the caste affiliations, have significant effects. Metros are not associated with higher prevalence rates.

TABLE 8.2 Tobit Analysis of Factors Associated with Average Incidence of NCDs—Urban India (2004–5)

Dependent Variable: Number of Household Members suffering divided by household size	No. of observations = 2610 LR Chi^2 (11) = 412.09 Prob>Chi2 = 0.0000					
	Coefficient			Elasticity		
Obesity Dummy (=0 if BMI of any member is less than 25, else = 1)	0.038	(3.87)	***	0.028	(3.87)	***
Female headed household	−0.011	(−0.53)	–	−0.001	(−0.53)	–
Age of household head	0.017	(6.23)	***	1.717	(6.25)	***
Age of household head – squared	0.000	(−5)	***	−0.660	(−5.02)	***
Highest education level of female adults	0.000	(−0.16)	–	−0.003	(−0.16)	–
Highest education level of male adults	−0.001	(−0.37)	–	−0.011	(−0.37)	–
Log of monthly per capita expenditure	0.169	(9.54)	***	0.287	(8.75)	***
Caste Dummy (SC)	−0.018	(−1.23)	**	−0.006	(−1.23)	**
Caste Dummy (ST)	−0.052	(−1.16)	**	−0.001	(−1.16)	**
Caste Dummy (OBC)	0.005	(0.43)	–	0.003	(0.43)	–
Dummy: Metro Areas = 1, Other Urban = 0	0.010	(0.91)	**	0.006	(0.91)	**
Constant	−1.612	(−13.15)				

Source: Authors' calculations based on IHDS, 2005.

Notes: Reference category for caste dummies: Others; ***, **, * denote significant at 1 per cent, 5 per cent, and 10 per cent, respectively.

Number of household members suffering from either high blood pressure, heart disease, diabetes, or cancer divided by household size.

As in the rural sample, highest elasticity is associated with age (net of that of age squared), followed by that of per capita expenditure, and overweight/obese adults.

ALL-INDIA

All-India results reveal a similar pattern, but with a few differences, as given in Table 8.3. Overweight/obese adults are associated with

TABLE 8.3 Tobit Analysis of Factors Associated with Average Incidence of NCDs—All India (2004–5)

Dependent Variable: Number of Household Members suffering divided by the household size	No. of observations = 6537 LR Chi^2 (12) = 809.79 Prob>Chi2 = 0.0000					
	Coefficient			Elasticity		
Obesity Dummy (=0 if BMI of any member is less than 25, else = 1)	0.066	(7.43)	***	0.025	(7.43)	***
Female headed household	−0.024	(−1.3)	**	−0.002	(−1.3)	**
Age of household head	0.015	(7.41)	***	1.293	(7.43)	***
Age of household head – squared	0.000	(−6.58)	***	−0.553	(−6.59)	***
Sector Dummy (Rural)	0.011	(1.17)	**	0.013	(1.17)	**
Sector Dummy (Metro Urban)	0.067	(5.5)	***	0.014	(5.51)	***
Highest education level of female adults	0.004	(3.99)	***	0.038	(4)	***
Highest education level of male adults	−0.003	(−2.68)	***	−0.038	(−2.67)	***
Log of monthly per capita expenditure	0.155	(11.72)	***	0.276	(11.58)	***
Caste Dummy (SC)	0.010	(0.95)	**	0.004	(0.95)	**
Caste Dummy (ST)	−0.058	(−2.29)	**	−0.004	(−2.29)	**
Caste Dummy (OBC)	0.005	(0.6)	–	0.004	(0.6)	–
Constant	−1.498	(−15.77)				

Source: Authors' calculations based on IHDS, 2005.
Notes: Reference category for sector dummies: Urban areas; Reference category for caste dummies: Others; ***, **, * denote significant at 1 per cent, 5 per cent, and 10 per cent, respectively.
Number of household members suffering from either high blood pressure, heart disease, diabetes, or cancer divided by household size.

higher prevalence of NCDs, as in the rural and urban samples; age has a positive relationship with this prevalence, but it weakens with advancing age; urban metros display higher prevalence; education of adult females has a positive effect, while that of adult males has a negative effect, as in the rural sample; per capita expenditure has a positive effect, as in both rural and urban samples; only ST households display lower prevalence of NCDs relative to 'others'.

Highest elasticity is associated with age net of that of its square; the next highest with respect to per capita expenditure; and much lower is the elasticity with respect to overweight/obese adults; metros display slightly higher prevalence compared to the remaining urban areas; and STs display negligibly lower elasticity relative to 'others'.

In sum, age and affluence emerge as key factors in determining the prevalence of NCDs. Somewhat surprising is the small effect of overweight and obesity.

Number of Ailments

So far, the focus was on the factors associated with average incidence of NCDs. A related but different measure of incidence of NCDs—in which number of ailments reported by an adult are added up and divided by household size—is used here. The results are given in Tables 8.4–8.6. As most of the results are similar to those in Tables 8.1–8.3, our comments are confined to the elasticities.

RURAL

Let us first consider the results in Table 8.4. Going by the absolute magnitude, the elasticity of number of NCDs with respect to age (net of that of its square) is highest, followed by that of per capita expenditure. Elasticities with respect to education of adult females and males are low. But somewhat surprisingly, elasticity of NCDs with respect to overweight/obese adults is even lower. Still lower are the elasticities with respect to SCs and STs.

URBAN

The highest (absolute) elasticity is with respect to age (net of that of its square), followed by that of per capita expenditure. In fact, it is larger than that in the rural sample. Consistent with earlier results, overweight/obesity has a small elasticity.

ALL INDIA

We refer here to the results in Table 8.6. As in the rural and urban samples, some of the results are similar, except that there are two

TABLE 8.4 Tobit Analysis of Factors Associated with Number of NCD Ailments Reported—Rural India (2004–5)

Dependent Variable: Number of ailments reported divided by the household size	No. of observations = 3927 LR Chi^2 (10) = 386.58 Prob>Chi2 = 0.0000					
	Coefficient			Elasticity		
Obesity Dummy (=0 if BMI of any member is less than 25, else = 1)	0.119	(6.68)	***	0.023	(6.72)	***
Female headed household	−0.046	(−1.25)	**	−0.002	(−1.25)	**
Age of household head	0.017	(4.53)	***	1.026	(4.54)	***
Age of household head – squared	0.000	(−4.3)	***	−0.472	(−4.31)	***
Highest education level of female adults	0.010	(4.85)	***	0.048	(4.88)	***
Highest education level of male adults	−0.006	(−3.19)	***	−0.050	(−3.18)	***
Log of monthly per capita expenditure	0.242	(9.43)	***	0.307	(9.33)	***
Caste Dummy (SC)	0.040	(2.05)	**	0.012	(2.05)	**
Caste Dummy (ST)	−0.083	(−1.95)	**	−0.005	(−1.96)	**
Caste Dummy (OBC)	0.004	(0.23)	–	0.002	(0.23)	–
Constant	−2.137	(−11.97)				

Source: Authors' calculations based on IHDS, 2005.

Notes: Reference category for caste dummies: Others; ***, **, * denote significant at 1 per cent, 5 per cent, and 10 per cent, respectively.

Number of NCD ailments reported by adults divided by household size.

dummies: one for rural households and another for metros (urban). The elasticities reveal a pattern not dissimilar from that observed in the rural and urban samples. Age net of the elasticity of age squared is highest, followed by that of expenditure. The elasticity with respect to overweight/obese adults is low. The lowest elasticity is with respect to ST affiliation.

TABLE 8.5 Tobit Analysis of Factors Associated with Number of NCD Ailments Reported—Urban India (2004–5)

Dependent Variable: Number of ailments reported divided by the household size	No. of observations = 2610 LR Chi^2 (11) = 388.39 Prob>Chi2 = 0.0000					
	Coefficient			Elasticity		
Obesity Dummy (=0 if BMI of any member is less than 25, else = 1)	0.049	(3.92)	***	0.029	(3.92)	***
Female headed household	−0.010	(−0.37)	–	−0.001	(−0.37)	–
Age of household head	0.020	(5.82)	***	1.595	(5.84)	***
Age of household head – squared	0.000	(−4.57)	***	−0.600	(−4.58)	***
Highest education level of female adults	0.000	(0.22)	–	0.005	(0.22)	–
Highest education level of male adults	−0.001	(−0.35)	–	−0.011	(−0.35)	–
Log of monthly per capita expenditure	0.197	(8.78)	***	0.334	8.67	***
Caste Dummy (SC)	−0.025	(−1.34)	**	−0.007	(−1.35)	**
Caste Dummy (ST)	−0.061	(−1.06)	**	−0.001	(−1.06)	**
Caste Dummy (OBC)	0.010	(0.76)	**	0.006	(0.76)	**
Dummy: Metro Areas = 1, Other Urban = 0	0.020	(1.43)	**	0.009	(1.43)	**
Constant	−1.917	(−12.35)				

Source: Authors' calculations based on IHDS, 2005.

Notes: Reference category for caste dummies: Others; ***, **, * denote significant at 1 per cent, 5 per cent, and 10 per cent respectively.

Number of NCD ailments reported by adults divided by household size.

In sum, there is robust confirmation of the important roles of ageing and affluence in determining the burden of NCDs, regardless of how it is measured. Overweight/obesity among adults, however, has a small but robust positive effect. That this is a consequence of selective reporting of BMI by adults cannot be ruled out.

TABLE 8.6 Tobit Analysis of Factors Associated with Number of NCD Ailments Reported –All India (2004–05)

Dependent Variable: Number of ailments reported divided by the household size	No. of observations = 6537 LR Chi^2 (12) = 828.13 Prob>Chi2 = 0.0000					
	Coefficient			Elasticity		
Obesity Dummy (=0 if BMI of any member is less than 25, else = 1)	0.075	(6.93)	***	0.023	(6.93)	***
Female headed household	−0.027	(−1.19)	**	−0.002	(−1.19)	**
Age of household head	0.018	(7.3)	***	1.274	(7.32)	***
Age of household head – squared	0.000	(−6.41)	***	−0.538	(−6.42)	***
Sector Dummy (Rural)	0.015	(1.34)	**	0.015	(1.34)	**
Sector Dummy (Metro Urban)	0.082	(5.51)	***	0.014	(5.52)	***
Highest education level of female adults	0.005	(4.32)	***	0.041	(4.33)	***
Highest education level of male adults	−0.004	(−2.83)	***	−0.040	(−2.83)	***
Log of monthly per capita expenditure	0.193	(11.97)	***	0.282	(11.83)	***
Caste Dummy (SC)	0.008	(0.6)	–	0.002	(0.6)	–
Caste Dummy (ST)	−0.074	(−2.38)	**	−0.004	(−2.39)	**
Caste Dummy (OBC)	0.003	(0.26)	–	0.002	(0.26)	–
Constant	−1.861	(−16.04)				

Source: Authors' calculations based on IHDS, 2005.
Notes: Reference category for sector dummies: Urban areas; Reference category for caste dummies: Others; ***, **, * denote significant at 1 per cent, 5 per cent, and 10 per cent respectively.
Number of NCD ailments reported by adults divided by household size.

***

Ageing, growing affluence of Indians, obesity, and higher prevalence rates of NCDs—especially CVD and diabetes—set the stage for the preceding analysis. As these diseases are associated with enormous economic burden on households and macro effects through lower savings, lower labour productivity, and growth decelerations, it is necessary to understand the underlying factors. Towards this objective, detailed analyses were carried out using different specifications of the burden of NCDs.

In one measure, the average refers to number of adults reporting suffering from any of the four NCDs divided by household size. In another, taking account of the fact that there are overlaps between various diseases (for example, between high blood pressure and heart disease), and some individuals report suffering from more than one ailment, we added up the different ailments reported by adult household members, and divided it by household size. As mostly similar results are obtained using both measures, a selective summary is given below.

Our analysis throws new light on the underlying factors, based on a recent nationwide household survey. Disaggregation of the sample into rural and urban, and a broad analytical framework encompassing household characteristics including age, whether any adult is overweight or obese, education, caste affiliations, per capita expenditure, and location—rural, urban, and metros—help unravel the links between them and NCDs, with a few surprises.

As the demographic transition advances, and the population ages without associated improvements in living conditions, nutrition, and better access to health services, it is not surprising that ageing is a key factor in the growing burden of NCDs. Affluence also has a significant role through lifestyle changes and dietary composition. As caste affiliation better captures aspects of non-monetary deprivation, those at the bottom of the caste hierarchy (STs) have much lower prevalence of these diseases. Somewhat surprising is the low effect of overweight/obesity on NCDs. This result has to be interpreted with caution, given the selective reporting of BMI by adults.

In conclusion, although the share of NCDs in the disease burden has risen, that of communicable diseases remains high, pointing to a 'double disease' burden. The shift of the disease burden toward NCDs will increase demand on the health care system. With more health care currently financed with private, out-of-pocket resources, it will be increasingly harder for households to escape poverty, while more will be driven into poverty. As rural population migrates to urban areas, the associated lifestyle changes are likely to elevate NCD risks. Extreme poverty and foetal and early childhood undernutrition, from both the current situation and past exposure, are likely to create a large pool of those at elevated risk.

ANNEXURE

TABLE **8A.1** Definitions of Variables Used

Variables	Definition
Dependent variables	
Average incidence of NCDs	= Number of household members suffering from either high blood pressure, heart disease, diabetes, or cancer divided by household size (range: 0 to 1)
Number of ailments per person	= Number of ailments reported by all adult household members/household size
Explanatory variables	
Obesity Dummy	= 0 if BMI of any member is less than 25, else = 1
Age	Age (years) of the household head
Square of age	Square of age
Gender	= 1 if head of the household is female; 0 if male
Highest education: Female	Number of years completed in education by most educated female in the household
Highest education: Male	Number of years completed in education by most educated male in the household
Other (reference)	= 1 if social group is other; 0 otherwise
SC	= 1 if social group is SC; 0 otherwise
ST	= 1 if social group is ST; 0 otherwise
OBC	= 1 if social group is OBC; 0 otherwise
Log PCME	Log of per capita monthly expenditure
Urban – Non-Metro (reference)	= 1 if urban area is a non-metro; 0 otherwise
Metro	= 1 if urban area is a metro; 0 otherwise
Rural	= 1 if rural area; 0 otherwise

Source: IHDS, 2005.

Note: For rural areas, PSU is a village, and, for urban areas, it is a town.

NOTES

1. NCDs include conditions such as cardio-vascular diseases (CVD), cancer, diabetes, chronic obstructive pulmonary disease (COPD), asthma, neuro-psychiatric conditions (mental disorders), eye conditions, skin diseases, diseases of the digestive system, and genitourinary conditions (prostate disorders), among others (Mahal *et al.* 2009).

2. Population ageing is the increase in the number and proportion of older people in society. Population ageing is due to migration, longer life expectancy (decreased death rate), and decreased birth rate.

3. Women who were malnourished as children are at increased risk of being centrally obese and having impaired glucose tolerance as adults. If these conditions affect a woman's pregnancy, her offspring will be at increased risk of early obesity and diabetes (Popkin *et al.* 2012).

4. Age-standardized undiscounted DALYs have been widely used to measure the burden of disease. These measure the number of years a person would lose due to disability and premature mortality. An advantage of using DALYs is that it considers years with disability, and thus includes conditions that, although not fatal, can be a large social and economic burden (World Bank 2011).

5. This draws upon World Bank (2011) and Mahal *et al.* (2009).

6. For a rigorous and innovative analysis of the overall effect of health on income, labour productivity, savings, and population effects, see Bloom *et al.* (2009).

7. This is a summary of the material provided by Sonal Desai, the principal author of IHDS.

8. 'I have disease Z'. If X = 1 when the response is 'yes', then we can decompose the probability into $P(X) = P(X|Z)*P(Z) + P(X|{\sim}Z)*P({\sim}Z)$. We are interested in measuring P(Z), but only observe P(X) having to contend with false negatives $P(X|Z) \neq 1$ generally from ignorance and misdiagnosis, or false positives $P(X|{\sim}Z) \neq 0$ from either misdiagnosis or hypochondria (Chaudhury *et al.* 2008).

9. Although BMI data are available for slightly younger population, for reasons of comparability, we have confined our analysis to the sub-sample >22 years.

10. It is widely believed that populations from South, East, and South-East Asia have a heightened susceptibility to diabetes when combined with unhealthy diets, low levels of physical activity, and smoking (Bajpai *et al.* 2010).

11. Often measurement of living standards in a money metric is problematic (because of the difficulties in measuring inputs and outputs that are not marketed). To overcome this difficulty, some proximate indicators (for example, caste and location) are also considered

12. The average poverty line is Rs 356 per person per month in rural areas (at 2004–5 prices), and Rs 538 in urban areas. State-wise poverty lines range from Rs 292 to Rs 478 in rural areas, and Rs 378 to Rs 668 in urban areas (Desai *et al.* 2010).
13. In principle, we should have computed the odds ratios. As some of the matrices are 3 × 3 (all NCDs have a separate category of cured), a multinomial logit model is appropriate. This, however, was not attempted as it is computationally tedious (Greene 2003).
14. Bajpai *et al.* (2010) draw attention to rapid spread of diabetes to rural areas.
15. This analysis is based on the IHDS 2005. Further details are available in Gaiha *et al.* (2009).
16. BMI = (weight in kg/height in m^2).
17. A WHO expert consultation reviewed the BMI cut-offs for overweight and obese in 2002. It concluded that Asians generally have a higher percentage of body fat than white people of the same age, sex, and BMI. Also, the proportion of Asian people with risk factors for type 2 diabetes and CVD is substantial even below the existing WHO BMI cut off point of 25kg/m^2. Thus, current WHO cut-off points do not provide an adequate basis for taking action on risks related to overweight and obesity in many Asian populations. However, the available data do not necessarily indicate one clear BMI cut-off point for all Asians for overweight or obese. The BMI cut-off point for observed risk in different Asian population varies from 22 kg/m^2 to 25kg/m^2; for high risk it varies from 26kg/m^2 to 31kg/m^2 (WHO 2004). So, while the consultation agreed on the need for revision, it refrained from recommending precise adjustments.
18. As the BMI sample is small, the results require cautious interpretation.
19. If the dependent variable is essentially continuous over strictly positive values but takes on zero with positive probability, using a standard regression model would give inconsistent and biased estimates. In such a case, the tobit specification gives a better estimation of the production function by ensuring non-negative predicted values for the dependent variable. For a formal exposition of the tobit specification, refer to Wooldridge (2006).
20. A health production function, akin to the production function, shows the relationship between outputs and inputs, where output refers to some measure of health status, and inputs include initial health status, nutrient intakes or food prices, incomes, demographic factors, and the health environment. For a clear exposition, see Behrman and Deolalikar (1988, 1990).
21. Note that the marginal effects differ from the tobit coefficients, but the sign is not affected (Wooldridge 2006).

22. While education and expenditure per capita are correlated, it does not necessarily follow that the collinearity between them is strong. The fact that education has a significant effect on the number of NCDs implies that the effect of the former is isolated. It is arguable, of course, that the effect is not as precise as desired.
23. As log of per capita expenditure and per capita expenditure are monotonically related, we use the latter for expositional convenience.

9 Food Subsidy, Income Transfer, and the Poor

*A Comparative Analysis of the Public Distribution System in India's States**

Raghbendra Jha, Raghav Gaiha,
Manoj K. Pandey, and Nidhi Kaicker

Although rapid economic growth in India has led to steady progress in reducing poverty, malnutrition remains widespread, and ensuring food access for the poor remains a priority for the government. Total food subsidy amounted to around 1 per cent of GDP in 2009. The largest food subsidy programme, the Targeted Public Distribution System (TPDS or PDS for short), provides households access to subsidized food staples (wheat, rice) and other items (edible oils, kerosene, sugar) (OECD 2011; Svedberg 2012). Further, the TPDS serves as a minimum support price mechanism for farmers. Other special programmes include the Mid-Day Meals Scheme (MDMS) which offers a hot meal to all children attending government-funded elementary schools.

Till 1992 the PDS was a general entitlement scheme for all consumers without any specific target. Although the food subsidy under the PDS was large, its effects on the poor were minimal (Radhakrishna and Subbarao 1997).[1] Their analysis of 1986–7 household data showed that per capita gains to rural consumers from all consumer subsidies

* Reprinted from *Journal of Policy Modeling*, vol. 35, no. 6, R. Jha, R. Gaiha, M.K. Pandey, and N. Kaicker, 'Food Subsidy, Income Transfer and the Poor: A Comparative Analysis of the Public Distribution System in India's States', pp. 887–908, June 2013, with permission from Elsevier Limited.

(food and non-food) were just Rs 2 per month, or 2.7 per cent of monthly per capita expenditures (MPCE). The effects, therefore, on poverty and nutrition were negligible. Before motivating this chapter, we briefly discuss the impact of TPDS on nutrition and poverty and diversions of TPDS stocks.

In response to the concern for reducing subsidies in view of the growing fiscal deficit, the government redesigned the PDS in 1997. The new programme, TPDS, aimed to reduce subsidies to the non-poor and enhance those to the poor. Its salient features (Bhalotra 2004; Jha and Ramaswami 2010; Kochar 2005; Planning Commission 2008; Svedberg 2012) are as follows.

TPDS distinguishes between households below the poverty line (BPL households) and those above the official state-specific poverty lines (APL). State governments are responsible for identifying BPL households, using multiple criteria including indicators such as land operated/owned, ownership of TVs, motorcycles, and other durables. Foodgrains are purchased by the central government, through the Food Corporation of India (FCI), at predetermined minimum support prices (MSP). The government determines a uniform central issue price at which foodgrains are sold by FCI to state governments for distribution through the TPDS. The TPDS initially fixed the BPL household entitlements at 10 kg of foodgrains per month, and gradually raised these to 35 kg. Since 2000–1, BPL households are entitled to purchase rice from fair price shops (FPS) for Rs 5.65 per kg and wheat for Rs 4.15. APL allocations varied across states and were calculated as the difference between the state's allocation of foodgrains and BPL allotments. State allocations are determined by the central government on the basis of last 10 years' average take-up of subsidized foodgrains. As market prices rose more than subsidized prices, there were substantial increases in BPL subsidies. In 2002, a new TPDS window was opened, Antyodaya Anna Yojana (AAY), under which the poorest of the poor were given the option to buy food at even more subsidized prices.[2] Prices for AAY households are Rs 3 per kg of rice and Rs 2 per kg of wheat, respectively.

TPDS, Nutrition, and Poverty

We provide below a selective review of recent, important contributions.

Kochar (2005) confirms a positive and significant but small effect of foodgrain subsidies on caloric intake. The elasticity of caloric intake to the foodgrain subsidy is 0.06, substantially lower than available estimates of the expenditure elasticity of caloric intake for low income households—an average of 0.3 (Strauss and Thomas 1995). Nevertheless, targeting should have raised the subsidy to the poor to a level to induce a substantially higher caloric intake. TPDS monthly wheat subsidy rose from Rs 7 per BPL household in 1993 to Rs 48 by April 2000. Assuming a slightly higher elasticity of 0.08, this 586 per cent increase in the TPDS subsidy should have raised the BPL caloric intake by 65 per cent. But the actual increase over the period 1993–7 was marginal, from 1933 calories to 1964 per person per day. This difference reflects the gap between TPDS purchases and entitlements, particularly among poor households. Over 1993–9, the value of foodgrain subsidies received by poor households fell from 15 per cent to 11 per cent of their entitlements, underscoring the point that a targeted programme that aims to enhance the benefits to the poor while restricting them to the non-poor, may adversely affect the off-take by the poor relative to the same entitlements to all under a universal programme.[3]

Kochar (2005) argues that the relationship between profits and the number of customers generates a profit maximizing level of procurement by FPS owners.[4] As the optimal amount of FPS procurement falls with a decline in the number of customers, the change to a targeted programme discourages them from holding TPDS stocks, thus limiting supply to BPL households. Kochar's empirical analysis compares a uniform policy that gives all households the same entitlement and a targeted policy that increases BPL entitlements, but at the expense of APL entitlements. The result confirms the superiority of the uniform policy in improving off-take by the poor, but ignores the issue of diversions from FPS to the open market. As argued below, nothing short of a drastic overhaul of the TPDS, but with the same outlay, has the potential of targeting benefits better to the poor. Universalizing the food subsidy is escapist and has feeble empirical support.

While BPL and AAY cardholders are allowed to buy 35 kg of subsidized grains per month, the actual purchase is just 14.7 kg in rural areas and 17.4 kg in urban areas (Svedberg 2012). According to the NSSO 2004–5 survey, only 37.6 per cent of rural households below the poverty line have BPL cards (the corresponding figure is 25.7 per cent for urban areas). The reasons for buying much lower amounts than entitled include, among others, long distances to an FPS, irregular availability of grains in these shops, participants not being allowed to buy grains in small instalments, low quality of grains offered, preference for local grain variety, and small difference between TPDS and market prices. Consequently, the actual subsidy received by the poor is extremely low—less than Rs 4 per kg (of foodgrains),[5] that is, about 12–15 per cent of what the income transfer would have been had the system been well targeted, and households purchased the entire ration allocated to them. Income boosts with TPDS are 1.4 per cent in rural areas and 0.9 per cent in urban areas, but had the system worked without flaws, the income boosts would have been 7.4 per cent and 5.4 per cent for rural and urban areas, respectively.

Based on NSS data for 2004–5, Svedberg (2012) shows that poverty impacts were considerably lower than potential; the estimated income gap was 20.2 per cent in both rural and urban areas, implying that MPCE for the average poor household fell short of the poverty line by 20.2 per cent. The reduction in income gap is about 1 per cent as a result of the TPDS subsidy, as against one-third of the actual gap had the system worked without any exclusionary error and full utilization of entitlements.

Leakages are substantial. More than one-third (36.7 per cent) of the subsidized grain intended for poor households ends up as sales to non-poor households. About 10 per cent of all grains are spoilt during storage and transportation. 58 per cent of the subsidized foodgrains do not reach BPL families because of identification errors, non-transparent operations, and unethical practices in the implementation of TPDS (Planning Commission 2008). Further, given the high cost of handling foodgrains, the government ends up spending Rs 8.5 to transfer Re 1 to the poor (Svedberg 2012).

Profitability, Corruption, and Diversion

For 388 households in eight villages of Rajasthan in 2002–3, Khera (2011) analyses profitability of FPS and forms of corruption at different stages, and diversion of PDS supplies to open markets. She shows that one-third of sample households in Rajasthan have access to the TPDS. Among those with access to the TPDS (the BPL households or BPL+AAY cardholders), utilization levels are low both in terms of proportion of households buying some grain from the TPDS as well as quantities purchased. Barely 13 per cent of BPL households availed of the full entitlement. Worse, about one-third of the households did not buy anything from TPDS. The average bought was 12.6 kg (as against an entitlement of 35 kg).

Estimates of diversion of TPDS supplies, based on comparison of off-take data from the Ministry of Food and Consumer Affairs, Government of India, and consumption data from NSS (61st round) are alarmingly high and reveal that two-fifths of the official TPDS off-take was diverted. Less than one-fifth of rice was diverted compared with more than two-thirds of wheat. There is also a clear North–South divide in these diversions. In mainly rice eating southern states, the proportion of foodgrains diverted ranged from 11–48 per cent. Wheat eating states concentrated in the north had diversions ranging from 43–88 per cent. Khera (2011) makes the unverified conjecture that there are within region variations as well, depending on how vociferous the consumers are.

Wheat diversions for FPS are very profitable. The shopkeeper gets a paltry margin of 7 paise per kg of wheat sold to a BPL household, as compared with a margin of Rs 1.97 for selling this amount in the open market, and a much higher margin of Rs 4.50 per kg of AAY wheat. An honest FPS earns no more than Rs 100 per month, while on certain assumptions of amounts diverted, the profit is Rs 7,972 (net of transportation costs). Hence, the incentive to cheat is irresistible.

Corruption is rampant in obtaining a licence; commissions are paid to FCI officials for expediting supplies; amounts supplied are frequently lower than recorded. BPL consumers are often turned away on grounds of inadequate supplies; quality sold is abysmal; and buying quotas in instalments is discouraged. Under TPDS, low margins are compounded by shrinkage of volumes.

Objective

Against this background, the objective of this chapter is to examine the reasons for low real income transfers (RIT) through TPDS in three states: Andhra Pradesh, Maharashtra, and Rajasthan. In line with the concerns distilled from recent literature, our analysis focuses on variation in RIT through subsidized wheat, rice, and sugar in these states.

These are associated with poverty status and demographic characteristics of households, transaction costs of buying from TPDS, food price subsidy, and (proximate) measures of supply constraints.

Another related objective is to assess the effect of PDS on nutritional deprivation. We carry out a comparative analysis of PDS and NREG (National Rural Employment Guarantee), on nutritional deprivation, including micronutrient deprivation.

This chapter briefly describes the data and methodology, presents results on the basic profile of TPDS in the chosen states, and provides estimates of subsidy implicit in the TPDS scheme. It provides results of the Tobit estimation, and reviews the case for a universal food subsidy. It assesses the PDS and NREG effects on nutritional deprivation and provides observations from a broad policy perspective.

DATA AND METHODOLOGY

We draw upon primary household data, collected during 2007–8, from three Indian states: Rajasthan, Andhra Pradesh, and Maharashtra. The sample survey was designed to be representative for the following reasons. First, a list of NREG districts was compiled for each state. From these districts, three were selected on the basis of probability proportional to size (in this case, rural population as reported in the 2001 Census) in the case of Rajasthan. In a similar manner, six districts were selected for each of Andhra Pradesh and Maharashtra. In the next step, in the case of Rajasthan, for example, three villages were randomly selected from each district, followed by a random selection of households. Twenty-five households were selected from each of twenty villages spread over three districts. In Andhra Pradesh and Maharashtra, these twenty-five villages were spread over six districts each. In each village, twenty households were randomly selected, giving us a sample of 500 households in each of the three states surveyed. Apart from household level information, individuals within households were also interviewed. The data includes information on caste, occupation, landholdings, household size, NREG participation, type of ration card, and TPDS participation. The number of individuals interviewed for Rajasthan, Andhra Pradesh, and Maharashtra were 2664, 2190, and 2270, respectively.

Definition and Methodology

TPDS price for village v for food item j (for example, wheat, rice, sugar), P_{vj}, is defined as

$$P_{vj} = \exp\left(\frac{\sum_{i=1}^{n} \alpha_{vij} \log P_{vij}}{\sum_{i=1}^{n} \alpha_{vij}}\right) \text{where}$$

α_{vij} = expenditure on food item j by household i of village v

$\sum_{i=1}^{n} \alpha_{vij}$ = total TPDS expenditure on food item j by all households in village v

P_{vij} = price per unit quantity paid by household i of village v on food item j under TPDS, and

n = number of households in village v.

Similarly we compute market price. We then compute the excess of market price over TPDS price for village v for food item j = (Market price –TPDS price) ★ 100/market price.

RIT through TPDS is computed separately for each of the three food commodities by computing the product (Market price–PDS price)$_{vij}$ × q_{vij}(=quantity of *jth* food item bought by *ith* household in village v under TPDS).

TPDS participation: A household is said to be participating in TPDS if it bought some quantities of rice or wheat or sugar from an FPS in 2007–8.

Stochastic dominance comparisons of MPCE of participants and non-participants are made by examining the cumulative distribution functions (CDF) of the MPCE. We also use cross-tabulations to understand the distribution of waiting times for TPDS grain as well as the distribution of subsidy on foodgrain bought through the TPDS scheme.

Tobit Analysis

In principle, a two-step Heckman procedure is appropriate. In the first step, a probit is estimated to assess the determinants of probability of participation in TPDS. In the next step, RIT through subsidized purchase of each of the three items under TPDS are regressed on factors associated with them. Our experiments with the Heckman procedure consistently yielded an insignificant λ (inverse Mills ratio), implying that RITs could be analysed without the sample selection correction.[6]

For households that do not buy under the TPDS, there are zero RIT through subsidized food. Hence a Tobit specification is appropriate to examine the determinants of RITs through wheat, rice, and sugar (Greene 2003); Chapter 8 provides a brief exposition. The marginal effect (slope) is based on the conditional expectation E $(y|y>0, \mathbf{x})$, where y is the dependent variable, and $\mathbf{x}$ is a vector of explanatory variables.[7]

Our specification of explanatory variables focuses on three sets of variables: one relates to the economic status of a household. As entitlements of foodgrains (wheat and rice) vary with whether a household is a BPL (including AAY) card holder, it would have been appropriate to use this characteristic as an explanatory variable. However, this posed a problem as most of those with access to the TPDS in Andhra Pradesh, for example, were in fact, BPL card holders. We decided to use land owned (an exclusionary criterion under BPL classification when ownership exceeds five acres) as a measure of a household's economic status. Another set of variables is demographic, comprising household size, and its composition (number of male and female adults).

A major factor influencing the demand for food and RIT is the price subsidy under TPDS. TPDS price of a food commodity divided by its open market price at the village level reflects the subsidy—the lower the TPDS price relative to the market price, the larger is the subsidy per unit bought. Whether subsidies on food complements (for example, rice and wheat in some parts of India) affect RIT is also examined.

Surprisingly, BPL households frequently buy amounts of foodgrains that are a small fraction of their entitlements. There are two reasons for this: (i) there are high transaction costs of buying from FPS because of long distances to FPS, and long waiting periods at these shops; and (ii) there are inadequate supplies at FPS, mainly due to diversion to open markets where the margins are much higher. To capture the adequacy of supply, Kochar (2005) used number of APL households. Given the higher margins, the larger the number, the greater is the incentive for FPS to hold larger stocks. As the APL numbers are small in our sample, we have used proportion of BPL households in the village population on the assumption that lower margins on sales to BPL households are likely to be compensated for by larger numbers. Another factor that could negatively impact supply is distance to the nearest town. The longer the distance, the greater is the likelihood of inadequate supply.

Further, gains from major anti-poverty interventions such as NREG are sensitive to inequality in the distribution of endowments (typically land) in rural areas. As greater inequality in land distribution is often associated with asymmetric power relations, a hypothesis verified here is whether RIT under TPDS are lower in villages with greater inequality. However, any scalar measure of inequality in a distribution is an oversimplification. The Gini coefficient of land distribution, for example, could be high where proportions of landless or near landless are high, or it could also be high where those owning moderate and large amounts of land are high. So the results may vary with different forms of inequality.[8]

TPDS IN ANDHRA PRADESH, MAHARASHTRA, AND RAJASTHAN

We now review basic characteristics of households participating in TPDS, transaction costs of buying from FPS, food price subsidies, and real income gains.

Household Characteristics

The shares of the Schedule Castes (SCs), Scheduled Tribes (STs), and Other Backward Castes (OBCs) in the total population are nearly equal in Rajasthan. In Andhra Pradesh, the share of OBCs in the total population (under 49 per cent) is the highest, followed by SCs (about 29 per cent) and STs (under 10 per cent). In Maharashtra, the share of the OBCs in the total population is the highest among the three states (about 51 per cent), with considerably lower, though nearly equal, shares of the SCs (about 13 per cent) and STs (about 15 per cent).

The share of poor households in the total population is the highest in Rajasthan (about 41 per cent), with the highest share of acutely poor (about 30 per cent); Andhra Pradesh and Maharashtra stood second and third in terms of share of poor households in respective populations, with nearly the same share (about 25 per cent), although the proportion of acutely poor is greater in Andhra Pradesh than in Maharashtra.[9]

The distribution of land across households also varies significantly across the three states. Andhra Pradesh has the highest share of landless households (nearly 44 per cent). The share of the landless is nearly equal in Rajasthan and Maharashtra. Maharashtra has the highest percentages of households in the category of owning more than five acres (about 16 per cent), whereas those of Andhra Pradesh and Rajasthan are almost equal (about 4 per cent).

The education level of the household head differs in these states. While the share of illiterate household heads is the highest (above 44 per cent) in Andhra Pradesh, it is the lowest in Maharashtra (under 28 per cent). Rajasthan comes in between, with 38 per cent of households with illiterate heads. It has the highest (above 12 per cent) share of household heads with secondary and higher education levels, as compared to Maharashtra (under 9 per cent) and Andhra Pradesh (under 6 per cent).

The distribution of household size also differs in these states. While nearly 60 per cent of households in Andhra Pradesh have less than five members, the shares of this group in Maharashtra and Rajasthan are about 53 per cent and 38 per cent, respectively. Rajasthan has the highest share of large households (more than eight members).

TPDS Participation

The proportion of households participating in the TPDS is the highest in Andhra Pradesh (92 per cent), followed by Maharashtra (78 per cent), and then Rajasthan (58 per cent). In Rajasthan, the share of STs is the highest among TPDS participants, while in Andhra Pradesh and Maharashtra, the share of OBCs is the highest.

Among households participating in the TPDS in all three states, shares of non-poor households are significantly higher than those of the poor, with the ratio of non-poor to poor participating households being 1.2 (for Rajasthan), 2.6 (for Maharashtra), and 2.7 (for Andhra Pradesh).

Andhra Pradesh had the highest share of landless among TPDS participants (nearly 46 per cent), followed by Maharashtra (about 40 per cent), and Rajasthan (34 per cent). While the share of participants declines with increase in land owned in both Rajasthan and Andhra Pradesh, it increases after the initial decline in Maharashtra.

Among households that participated in the TPDS, the share of those with illiterate heads is nearly equal in Rajasthan and Andhra Pradesh (about 43–6 per cent), and it is lowest in Maharashtra (30 per cent). Further, while in Andhra Pradesh the share of household participating in the TPDS falls with higher level of education of the household head, in Rajasthan this declines till secondary education and then rises at the highest education level. In Maharashtra, this first increases (up to primary level) and then declines.

TPDS participation and household size reveal an interesting pattern. While in Andhra Pradesh and Maharashtra small households (with ≤4 members) exhibit highest share of TPDS participation, in Rajasthan relatively large households (5–8 members) do so.

Excess of Market Price over TPDS Price—Extent of Subsidy

To assess the difference between subsidized food price and market price, we computed excess of market price over PDS price for wheat, rice, and sugar at the village level.[10] Our key observations, based on Table 9.1, are as follows:

In the case of wheat in Rajasthan, the excess of market price over TPDS price varies in the range of 50 per cent to 90 per cent, with the highest concentration of villages (about 57 per cent) in the range 60–70 per cent. In Maharashtra, the excess of market price over TPDS price varies in the range 40 per cent to 90 per cent, with about 88 per cent of villages in the range 40–70 per cent.

In the case of rice, the minimum range of excess of market price over TPDS price is 30–50 per cent in all three states. While in Rajasthan and Maharashtra very small concentrations of villages are found in the highest range of price differences of 80–90 per cent and 70–80 per cent, in Andhra Pradesh, about 28 per cent of the villages are concentrated in the highest range (80–90 per cent). However, in all three states, the majority of the villages have excess of market price over TPDS price in the range of 50–70 per cent.

TABLE 9.1 Distribution of Excess of Market Price over PDS Price for Wheat, Rice, and Sugar Commodities

Ranges of excess of market price over PDS price	% of villages corresponding to commodity		
	Wheat	Rice	Sugar
Rajasthan			
0–10%	0.00	0.00	0.00
10–20%	0.00	0.00	6.25
20–30%	0.00	0.00	68.75
30–40%	0.00	5.26	18.75
40–50%	0.00	15.79	6.25
50–60%	21.74	31.58	0.00
60–70%	56.52	26.32	0.00
70–80%	13.04	15.79	0.00
80–90%	8.70	5.26	0.00
90–100%	0.00	0.00	0.00
Total number of villages for which information is available	*23*	*19*	*16*
Andhra Pradesh			
0–10%		0.00	8.00
10–20%		0.00	68.00
20–30%		0.00	16.00
30–40%		0.00	8.00
40–50%	*	4.00	0.00
50–60%		28.00	0.00
60–70%		36.00	0.00
70–80%		4.00	0.00
80–90%		28.00	0.00
90–100%		0.00	0.00
Total number of villages for which information is available	*1*	*25*	*25*

(continued)

TABLE 9.1 Continued

Ranges of excess of market price over PDS price	% of villages corresponding to commodity		
	Wheat	Rice	Sugar
Maharashtra			
0–10%	0.00	0.00	
10–20%	0.00	0.00	
20–30%	0.00	0.00	
30–40%	0.00	8.00	
40–50%	12.00	20.00	**
50–60%	44.00	32.00	
60–70%	32.00	28.00	
70–80%	8.00	12.00	
80–90%	4.00	0.00	
90–100%	0.00	0.00	
Total number of villages for which information is available	*25*	*25*	*0*

Source: Calculations based on primary data collected by R. Jha and R. Gaiha in 2007–8, from three Indian states, Rajasthan, Andhra Pradesh, and Maharashtra.
Note: Details available on request.
* Data are available only for one village. ** Data are not available for any village.

For sugar, data on TPDS prices are available only for Rajasthan and Andhra Pradesh. In Rajasthan, nearly 69 per cent of villages have 20–30 per cent of excess of market price over TPDS price; in Andhra Pradesh, by contrast, the majority of villages (68 per cent) are concentrated in the excess range of 10–20 per cent.

Participation in TPDS by Income Class

To examine participation in TPDS by income class we study the cumulative distribution functions (CDF) of MPCE for participants and non-participants in TPDS (Figure 9.1), using stochastic dominance tests. The advantage of these tests is that inferences about targeting of the TPDS can be drawn over a permissible range of poverty cut-off points and for the Foster-Greer-Thorbecke (FGT) class of poverty indices.[11]

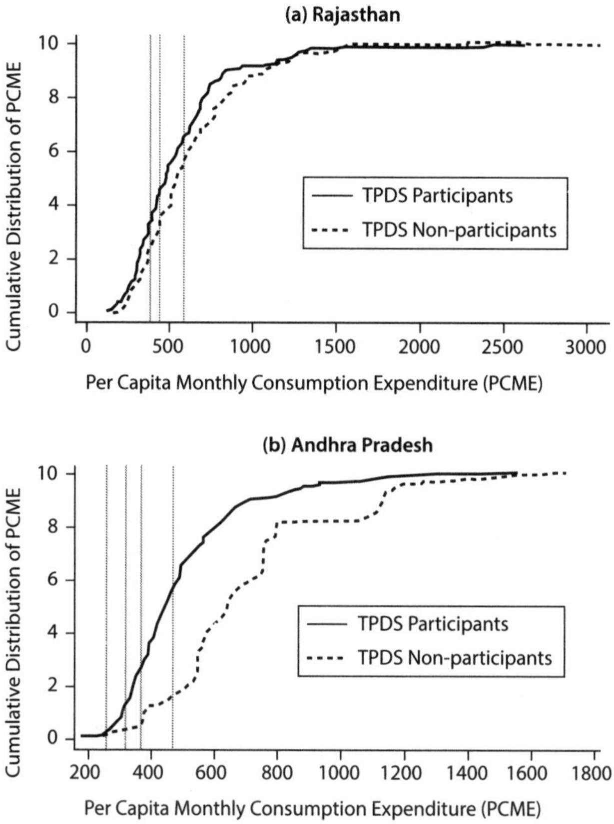

FIGURE 9.1 Cumulative Distribution Functions of Per Capita Monthly Consumption Expenditure for TPDS Participating and Non-participating Households

Source: Calculations based on primary data collected by R. Jha and R. Gaiha in 2007–8, from three Indian states, Rajasthan, Andhra Pradesh, and Maharashtra. Details available on request.

Notes: (a) Vertical reference lines are drawn at 383, 450 (poverty cut-off: Rs/person/month), and 585, respectively.

(b) Vertical reference lines are drawn at 239, 299, 352 (poverty cut-off: Rs/person/month) and 458, respectively.

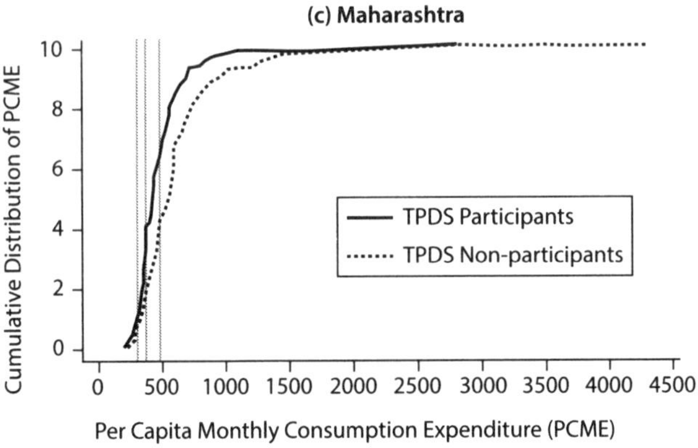

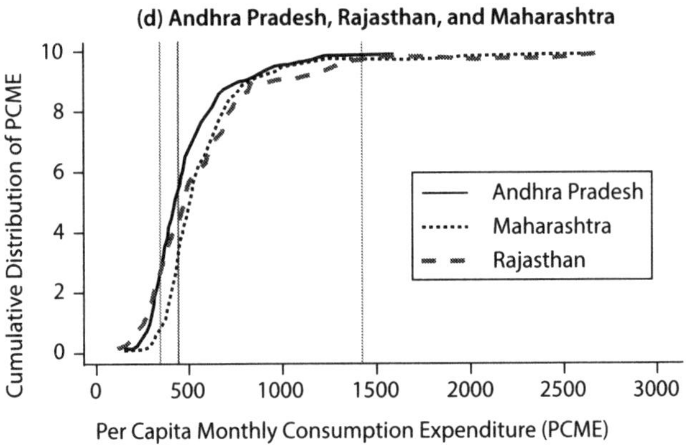

FIGURE 9.1 Continued

Notes: (c) Vertical reference lines are drawn at 371, 436 (poverty cut-off: Rs/person/month) and 567, respectively.

(d) Note:Vertical reference lines are drawn at poverty cut-offs for Andhra Pradesh (Rs 352/person/month), Maharashtra (Rs 436/person/month), Rajasthan (Rs 450/person/month), and 1400, respectively.

If, for example, the CDF of non-participants in TPDS lies below that of the participants over the permissible range of poverty cut-off points, the latter displays first order stochastic dominance (FOD). In that case, TPDS is better targeted on the poor in terms of all FGT poverty indices.

As the CDF of non-participants lies below that of participants over the PCME range, Rs ≥585, it follows that the latter FOD the former.[12] This implies that TPDS participants are poorer in terms of the FGT class of indices.

For Andhra Pradesh, there is robust confirmation of TPDS targeting in terms of the FGT class of poverty indices. Maharashtra also exhibits FOD of the CDF of non-participants over the CDF of participants, implying that the TPDS participants were poorer than non-participants in terms of the FGT indices. Comparisons of TPDS targeting across Rajasthan, Andhra Pradesh, and Maharashtra are, however, rendered difficult by the intersection of the CDFs of participants in Andhra Pradesh and Rajasthan within the permissible range, implying that FOD is ruled out. Given the overlap in the CDFs, what could be inferred is that targeting of the TPDS in these states is largely similar. However, as the CDF of participants for Maharashtra FOD the other CDFs, it follows TPDS was worst targeted in this state. Over a wide range of MPCE, both Andhra Pradesh and Rajasthan show FOD of the CDF of TPDS participants over that of the corresponding CDF for Maharashtra. So, in both Andhra Pradesh and Rajasthan, TPDS is better targeted than in Maharashtra. However, given that CDF of MPCE of participating households of Andhra Pradesh crosses over that of Rajasthan at the lower limit of the poverty cut-off point, and lies above it over the admissible poverty range, TPDS in Andhra Pradesh is better targeted than in Rajasthan.

Transaction Costs of Buying from Fair Price Shops (FPS)

We now examine transaction costs associated with buying from FPS. Key elements of transactions costs are the distance travelled to FPS and the waiting time to buy from these shops. Table 9.2 reports on distance to nearest FPS.

The range of distance of FPS from the household is highest for Rajasthan (0–12 km), followed by Andhra Pradesh and Maharashtra,

TABLE 9.2 Distribution of Distance from PDS Participating Households to Fair Price Shop

	Per cent of PDS participant households in		
	Rajasthan	Andhra Pradesh	Maharashtra
(a) PDS participating households to Fair Price Shop (km)			
0–1 km	35.60	71.99	84.24
1–2 km	27.93	18.32	02.12
2–3 km	13.51	7.81	07.55
3 km and above	22.95	1.88	06.10
All	*100.00*	*100.00*	*100.00*
(b) Distance from household to Fair Price Shop (km): Key Statistics			
Mean	1.58	0.64	0.39
Median	1.00	0.50	0.00
Standard deviation	1.64	0.62	0.89
Min	0.00	0.00	0.00
Max	12.00	3.00	3.00

Source: Calculations based on primary data collected by R. Jha and R. Gaiha in 2007–8, from three Indian states, Rajasthan, Andhra Pradesh, and Maharashtra.
Note: Details available on request.

with an almost equal range of 0–3 km. The average distance between a household and the FPS is the highest for Rajasthan, followed by Andhra Pradesh, and then Maharashtra. In Maharashtra, an overwhelming majority of the households (above 85 per cent) live within a range of 1 km from the FPS. The corresponding figures for Andhra Pradesh and Rajasthan are 72 per cent and 36 per cent, respectively.

As the distance to the FPS rises, the proportions of households in total population within specified intervals fall. Maharashtra, however, is an exception as the lowest proportion of households (under 2 per cent) live in the range 1–2 km.

In Table 9.3, we examine the distribution of waiting times for households participating in TPDS. In Rajasthan, about 45 per cent of the participating households had to wait for more than forty-five minutes to make purchases from FPS. By contrast, nearly 90 per cent of the

TPDS participants in Andhra Pradesh and 96 per cent in Maharashtra had to wait forty-five minutes or less at the FPS.

The mean waiting time for a TPDS participating household at FPS is highest in Rajasthan (more than sixty-four minutes), followed by Andhra Pradesh (about thirty minutes), and Maharashtra (about twenty-four minutes). There are variations in the mean waiting time among APL, BPL, and AAY households. In Rajasthan, BPL cardholders had the highest (mean) waiting time at the shop while APL card holders had the lowest. In Andhra Pradesh, APL card holders had the lowest mean waiting time, followed by BPL and AAY cardholders. In Maharashtra, BPL cardholders had the highest mean waiting time, followed by APL and AAY cardholders.

Other elements of transaction costs include defrauding by short-weight of foodgrains and inferior quality of grain supplied. In Rajasthan (Maharashtra), 20 per cent (14 per cent) of the reporting households believe that fair price shops short-weigh foodgrains. In Andhra Pradesh, a large proportion of households (32 per cent) believe that FPSs short-weigh grains. About 45 per cent of households in Rajasthan, 33 per cent in Maharashtra, and 70 per cent in Andhra Pradesh are satisfied with the quality of foodgrains.

Share of Expenditure on Food Bought from TPDS

Since entitlements for and participation of households in TPDS depend on whether the household has a BPL card, we now examine how BPL cards are distributed.

In Rajasthan, 30 per cent (6 per cent) of the households possessed a BPL (AAY) card. The corresponding figures were 19 per cent (5 per cent) among the non-poor households, and 44 per cent (8 per cent) among the poor households. In Maharashtra, 52 per cent (4 per cent) of the households possessed a BPL (AAY) card. The corresponding figure was 43 per cent (4 per cent) among the non-poor households, and 78 per cent (3.5 per cent) among the poor households. In Andhra Pradesh, 80 per cent (10 per cent) of the households possessed a BPL (AAY) card. The corresponding figure was 79 per cent (9 per cent) among the non-poor households, and 82 per cent (14 per cent) among the poor households.

TABLE 9.3 Distribution of Waiting Times for PDS Participating Households by Ration Card Type

Ranges of waiting times at the fair price shop (in minutes)	Per cent of PDS participant households by households are allotted				
	BPL	APL	Antyodaya	Others	All
Rajasthan					
≥0– ≤15	50.49 (17.60)	40.99 (24.91)	08.52 (14.72)	0.00	19.63
>15–≤30	40.90 (22.28)	49.92 (47.40)	09.18 (24.80)	0.00	30.68
>30–≤45	60.71 (05.54)	16.33 (02.60)	22.96 (10.38)	0.00	05.14
>45–≤60	49.92 (15.12)	28.58 (15.09)	21.50 (32.29)	0.00	17.06
>60	80.88 (39.46)	11.76 (10.00)	07.36 (17.81)	0.00	27.48
All	*56.33 (100.00)*	*32.31 (100.00)*	*11.36 (100.00)*	*0.00*	*100.00*
Andhra Pradesh					
≥0– ≤15	74.57 (11.60)	03.39 (25.82)	22.04 (26.85)	0.00 (0.00)	13.48
>15–≤30	88.22 (71.64)	01.87 (74.18)	09.19 (58.43)	0.72 (100.00)	70.37
>30–≤45	91.55 (06.88)	0.00 (0.00)	08.45 (04.97)	0.00 (0.00)	06.51

>45–≤60	98.67 (09.42)	0.00 (0.00)	01.33 (01.00)	0.00 (0.00)	08.28
>60	28.91 (0.45)	0.00 (0.00)	71.09 (08.75)	0.00 (0.00)	01.36
All	*86.65 (100.00)*	*1.77 (100.00)*	*11.07 (100.00)*	*0.51 (100.00)*	*100.00*
Maharashtra					
≥0– ≤15	58.75 (31.42)	32.31 (41.81)	08.94 (61.60)	0.00	35.87
>15–≤30	67.56 (44.67)	28.28 (45.26)	04.16 (35.47)	0.00	44.35
>30–≤45	79.66 (20.84)	19.47 (12.33)	0.87 (02.92)	0.00	17.55
>45–≤60	91.97 (02.83)	08.03 (0.60)	0.00 (0.00)	0.00	02.06
>60	100.00 (0.25)	0.00 (0.00)	0.00 (0.00)	0.00	0.17
All	*67.08(100.00)*	*27.72 (100.00)*	*05.20 (100.00)*	*0.00*	*100.00*

Source: Calculations based on primary data collected by R. Jha and R. Gaiha in 2007–8, from three Indian states, Rajasthan, Andhra Pradesh, and Maharashtra.

Note: Details available on request. Figures in parenthesis are the column percentages.

In Table 9.4 we give the distributions of the share of expenditure on food items bought from TPDS by participating households.

In the case of wheat, 59 per cent of participating households in Maharashtra bought 100 per cent of their wheat through FPS, and 34 per cent bought none. In Rajasthan, 20 per cent of the participating households bought 100 per cent of their wheat from FPS, and 48 per cent bought none.

In the case of rice, 35 per cent of households in Rajasthan made 100 per cent of their purchases through TPDS. The corresponding figures for Maharashtra and Andhra Pradesh were 55 per cent and 1.3 per cent, respectively. This suggests that households in Andhra Pradesh are more dependent on the market than on TPDS. About 58 per cent of households in Andhra Pradesh bought 12 per cent of their rice through TPDS. It is noteworthy that 63 per cent of the participating households in Rajasthan and 33 per cent in Maharashtra did not buy any rice from FPS. Mean share percentage of rice is the lowest in Andhra Pradesh (only 20 per cent). Maharashtra has the highest mean share (59 per cent), somewhat higher than Rajasthan (36 per cent).

In the case of sugar in Rajasthan, 22 per cent of the households bought 100 per cent of their sugar from FPS. The corresponding figure for Andhra Pradesh is about 41 per cent. 72 per cent of the participating households in Rajasthan and 33 per cent in Andhra Pradesh did not buy sugar from the TPDS. Mean share percentage of sugar is much higher in Andhra Pradesh (about 50 per cent) than in Rajasthan (about 26 per cent).

In Table 9.5, we report mean RIT from sales of various food items (wheat, rice and sugar) through TPDS per participating household per month.[13]

The mean RIT from wheat among participating households is highest in Rajasthan (Rs 93) and lowest in Maharashtra (Rs 60). Sufficient data are not available for Andhra Pradesh. In Rajasthan, RIT from TPDS for wheat to half of the participating households is Rs 100 or less (about 48 per cent of households have no RIT from TPDS), about 28 per cent have between Rs 100 and Rs 200, and 19 per cent have more than Rs 200. In Maharashtra about 34 per cent of the households had no RIT, and about 20 per cent had RIT of greater than Rs 100.

For wheat, it is interesting to note that mean RIT among the acutely poor households (Rs 56) is lower than that among moderately

TABLE 9.4 Distribution of Share of Expenditure on Food Items Bought from PDS among PDS Participating Households

Share (%)	Rajasthan		Andhra Pradesh		Maharashtra	
	Mean (%)	% PDS participating households	Mean (%)	% PDS participating households	Mean (%)	% PDS participating households
Share of wheat expenditure bought from PDS						
0	0.00	47.50			0.00	34.02
>0–≤20	16.00	9.50			16.17	0.97
>20–≤40	30.22	17.66			33.36	3.32
>40–≤60	51.98	4.42	NA	NA	58.44	1.76
>60–≤80	63.75	1.32			70.06	1.24
>80–≤100	100.00	19.61			100.00	58.69
All	*29.60*	*100.00*			*61.85*	*100.00*
Share of rice expenditure bought from PDS						
0	0.00	63.03	0.00	3.21	0.00	32.72
>0–≤20	14.29	0.94	11.99	57.96	14.57	1.09
>20–≤40	0.00	0.00	27.33	30.96	32.37	7.43
>40–≤60	47.73	0.75	45.56	5.68	47.67	3.29
>60–≤80	72.92	0.38	62.65	0.85	60.47	0.38
>80–≤100	100.00	34.89	100.00	1.34	100.00	55.09
All	*35.66*	*100.00*	*19.87*	*100.00*	*59.45*	*100.00*

(continued)

TABLE 9.4 Continued

Share (%)	Rajasthan		Andhra Pradesh		Maharashtra	
	Mean (%)	% PDS participating households	Mean (%)	% PDS participating households	Mean (%)	% PDS participating households
Share of sugar expenditure bought from PDS						
0	0.00	71.77	0.00	32.52		
>0–≤20	12.07	0.16	17.03	1.30		
>20–≤40	30.51	0.36	26.43	10.91		
>40–≤60	55.03	1.80	45.10	14.29	NA	NA
>60–≤80	67.64	3.99	63.64	0.15		
>80–≤100	100.00	21.93	100.00	40.84		
All	*25.74*	*100.00*	*50.48*	*100.00*		

Source: Calculations based on primary data collected by R. Jha and R. Gaiha in 2007–8, from three Indian states, Rajasthan, Andhra Pradesh, and Maharashtra.

Note: Details available on request.

TABLE 9.5 Distribution of Real Income Transferred (RIT) from PDS among Participating Households

Ranges of RIT from PDS (Rs) for different commodities	Rajasthan		Andhra Pradesh		Maharashtra	
	Mean	% of households	Mean	% of households	Mean	% of households
Wheat						
0	0.00	47.50			0.00	34.02
>0–≤50	–	0.00			36.85	15.89
>50–≤100	66.12	5.10			74.33	27.85
>100–≤150	127.41	20.85	NA	NA	124.69	11.96
>150–≤200	177.01	7.61			161.21	6.55
>200	263.33	18.94			221.96	3.72
All	*93.28*	*100.00*			*60.30*	*100.00*
Rice						
0	0.00	63.03	0.00	3.21	0.00	32.72
>0–≤50	30.28	13.42	39.32	2.49	34.18	29.65
>50–≤100	69.65	18.89	77.34	18.47	68.39	21.33
>100–≤150	124.19	3.08	123.83	31.37	137.29	7.28

(continued)

TABLE 9.5 Continued

Ranges of RIT from PDS (Rs) for different commodities	Rajasthan		Andhra Pradesh		Maharashtra	
	Mean	% of households	Mean	% of households	Mean	% of households
>150–≤200	181.57	0.77	162.14	27.01	181.20	3.70
>200	285.32	0.81	253.57	17.46	238.95	5.32
All	*24.75*	*100.00*	*142.17*	*100.00*	*54.12*	*100.00*
Sugar						
0	0.00	71.77	0.00	32.52		
>0–≤50	12.78	28.23	3.50	67.48		
>50–≤100	–	0.00	–	0.00		
>100–≤150	–	0.00	–	0.00	NA	NA
>150–≤200	–	0.00	–	0.00		
>200	–	0.00	–	0.00		
All	*3.61*	*100.00*	*2.36*	*100.00*		

Source: Calculations based on primary data collected by R. Jha and R. Gaiha in 2007–8, from three Indian states, Rajasthan, Andhra Pradesh, and Maharashtra.

Note: Details available on request.

poor (Rs 121) and non-poor (Rs 71 for moderately non-poor and Rs 128 for the relatively affluent) in Rajasthan; the RIT among the acutely poor (Rs 65) is slightly higher than in other categories (Rs 55 among moderately poor and Rs 58 among moderately non-poor) in Maharashtra.

Mean RIT for participating households from TPDS rice consumption is highest in Andhra Pradesh (Rs 142), followed by Maharashtra (Rs 54), and Rajasthan (Rs 25). In Rajasthan, about 63 per cent of participating households have no RIT from TPDS rice, and about 32 per cent have mean RIT of Rs 100 or less. In Andhra Pradesh, about 80 per cent participating households got mean RIT of more than Rs 100. In Maharashtra, only 16 per cent households obtained mean RIT of more than Rs 100 from rice consumption from TPDS; 33 per cent obtained no RIT, and 50 per cent had RIT of less than Rs 100.

For rice, mean RIT for acutely poor households is the lowest (Rs 14) in Rajasthan. In Andhra Pradesh, mean RIT is higher among the poor (Rs 167) than among the moderately non-poor (Rs 145) and relatively affluent (Rs 125). The opposite is true in Maharashtra, where the relatively affluent households have the highest mean RIT for rice (Rs 65 as compared with Rs 49 for the acutely poor).

Data for sugar is available only for Rajasthan and Andhra Pradesh. Mean RIT among participating households from sugar under TPDS

TABLE 9.6 Definition of Different Levels of Poverty

Levels of poverty	Rajasthan	Andhra Pradesh	Maharashtra
Acute poverty	If MPCE <Rs 383	If MPCE <Rs 299	If MPCE <Rs 371
Moderate poverty	If MPCE >= 383 but <Rs 450	If MPCE >= Rs 299 but <Rs 352	If MPCE >= Rs 371 but <Rs 436
Moderate Non-poverty	If MPCE >= Rs 450 but <Rs 585	If MPCE >= Rs 352 but <Rs 458	If MPCE >= Rs 436 but <Rs 567
Affluent	If MPCE >= Rs 585	If MPCE >= Rs 458	If MPCE >= Rs 567

Source: Authors' calculations based on Sen and Himanshu (2004).

in Rajasthan and Andhra Pradesh are Rs 4 and Rs 2 respectively. There is no clear pattern in mean RIT across participating households of different poverty status. Mean RITs per participating household from sugar consumption under TPDS is highest (Rs 13) in Rajasthan, and lowest (Rs 4) in Andhra Pradesh.

RESULTS ON TOBIT ESTIMATION

The results of the Tobit estimation are given in Tables 9.7a to 9.7g.

Andhra Pradesh

We first consider the association between economic status and RIT through subsidized rice, as reflected in the coefficients of land owned and its square (recall that land ownership results in exclusion from

TABLE 9.7a Results of Tobit Estimation (Andhra Pradesh—Sugar)

No. of Observations = 470 LR-chi2(10) = 116.64 Log Likelihood = −982.18 Andhra Pradesh – SUGAR	Prob>Chi-2 = 0.000 Pseudo R2 = 0.056			
	Coefficient			Marginal Effect
Land Owned	0.529	(1.48)	–	0.249
Square of Land Owned	−0.222	(−2.36)	★★	−0.104
Land Gini	2.202	(1.26)	–	1.034
Ratio of PDS to Market Price (Sugar)	−20.853	(−9.32)	★★★	−9.794
Distance to FPS	0.196	(0.71)	–	0.092
HH Size	0.230	(0.53)	–	0.108
HH Size – Squared	−0.011	(−0.25)	–	−0.005
No. of Adult Males	−0.143	(−0.61)	–	−0.067
No. of Adult Females	0.270	(1.09)	–	0.127
Distance to Nearest Town	−0.040	(−2.32)	★★	−0.019
Constant	17.401	(7.45)		
Sigma	*3.307*			
Left Censored Observations	*160*			
Uncensored Observations	*310*			

TABLE 9.7b Results of Tobit Estimation (Andhra Pradesh—Rice)

No. of Observations = 470 Prob>Chi-2 = 0.000
LR-chi2(11) = 205.54 Pseudo R2 = 0.039
Log Likelihood = −2543.32
Andhra Pradesh – RICE

	Coefficient			Marginal Effect
Land Owned	−13.971	(−3.59)	***	−13.146
Square of Land Owned	0.643	(1.3)	–	0.605
Land Gini	−66.077	(−2.2)	**	−62.178
Ratio of PDS to Market Price (Rice)	−201.705	(−7.39)	***	−189.804
Distance to FPS	−5.172	(−1.03)	–	−4.867
HH Size	43.947	(6.1)	***	41.354
HH Size – Squared	−2.767	(−3.75)	***	−2.604
No. of Adult Males	2.842	(0.71)	–	2.674
No. of Adult Females	1.514	(0.36)	–	1.425
Distance to Nearest Town	−3.632	(−4.25)	***	−3.418
Distance to Nearest Town – Squared	0.087	(5.59)	***	0.082
Constant	147.393	(4.62)		
Sigma	*58.723*			
Left Censored Observations	*22*			
Uncensored Observations	*448*			

BPL classification). The coefficient of land owned is negative and significant while that of land owned squared is not significant. So the poorer a household, the greater was the RIT. The effect of the land Gini is negative, implying that benefits were lower in villages with higher inequality in land distribution, possibly because there is greater diversion of rice to open markets from such villages. The lower the ratio of TPDS to market price of rice, the greater was RIT (either because the quantity bought was higher, or the same quantity bought translated into higher income gain because of a higher price subsidy). Distance to FPS shops, however, did not influence RIT as these shops were well dispersed. Household size, as expected, had a significant positive effect through higher rice demand, but the effect weakened among larger households. But the overall positive effect on RIT is substantial. As already indicated, with shift to TPDS and extremely

TABLE 9.7c Results of Tobit Estimation (Rajasthan—Wheat)

No. of Observations = 360 LR-chi2(12) = 58.32 Log Likelihood = −926.46 Rajasthan – WHEAT	Prob>Chi-2 = 0.000 Pseudo R2 = 0.031			
	Coefficient			Marginal Effect
Land Owned	67.007	(2.72)	***	19.640
Square of Land Owned	−6.380	(−2.03)	**	−1.870
Land Gini	334.294	(1.94)	*	97.982
Proportion of BPL Cardholders in a Village	726.659	(3.76)	***	212.984
Ratio of PDS to Market Price (Wheat)	−617.255	(−2.01)	**	−180.918
Ratio of PDS to Market Price (Rice)	249.268	(1.22)	–	73.061
Distance to FPS	−19.989	(−2.04)	**	−5.859
HH Size	−14.817	(−0.57)	–	−4.343
HH Size – Squared	0.846	(0.41)	–	0.248
No. of Adult Males	−19.217	(−0.96)	–	−5.632
No. of Adult Females	−12.782	(−0.58)	–	−3.746
Agricultural Wage Rate	3.374	(1.35)	–	0.989
Constant	−487.819	(−2.8)		
Sigma	*218.881*			
Left Censored Observations	*245*			
Uncensored Observations	*115*			

low margins on sales to BPL households, FPS have a weak incentive to maintain adequate stocks, or when the stocks are adequate, large supplies are diverted to the open market at much higher margins. Our data do not allow us to capture supply shortages or diversions to open markets (within or outside the village). A proxy variable—distance to the nearest town—is used on the premise that the longer the distance, the greater the probability that shortages will persist longer. Our results confirm this. The coefficient of distance to nearest town is negative and that of its square is positive. But altogether the effect is negative, implying that real incomes are more constrained in villages in far flung areas.

TABLE 9.7d Results of Tobit Estimation (Rajasthan—Rice)

No. of Observations = 360
LR-chi2(14) = 75.29
Log Likelihood = −617.84
Rajasthan – RICE

Prob>Chi-2 = 0.000
Pseudo R2 = 0.057

	Coefficient			Marginal Effect
Land Owned	21.654	(1.7)	*	5.248
Square of Land Owned	−1.364	(−0.9)	–	−0.330
Land Gini	102.801	(1.11)	–	24.913
Proportion of BPL Cardholders in a Village	341.053	(2.97)	***	82.650
Ratio of PDS to Market Price (Wheat)	−2,428.399	(−2.65)	***	−588.495
Price Ratio (Wheat) – Squared	3,706.375	(2.52)	**	898.198
Ratio of PDS to Market Price (Rice)	−759.773	(−1.53)	–	−184.123
Price Ratio (Rice) Squared	950.030	(1.74)	*	230.229
Distance to FPS	−7.294	(−1.41)	–	−1.768
HH Size	−15.957	(−1.21)	–	−3.867
HH Size – Squared	1.119	(1.07)	–	0.271
No. of Adult Males	−13.105	(−1.19)	–	−3.176
No. of Adult Females	−16.545	(−1.4)	–	−4.009
Agricultural Wage Rate	2.742	(1.97)	**	0.665
Constant	192.815	(1.01)		
Sigma	*105.363*			
Left Censored Observations	*278*			
Uncensored Observations	*82*			

RIT through subsidized sugar is positively linked to land owned—while the coefficient of land owned is positive and weakly significant, that of its square is negative and significant. The effect, however, is small. The land Gini is insignificant. The ratio of PDS to market price is negative and significant, suggesting that RITs are larger when the price subsidy is larger. The column of marginal effects indicates that price subsidy is key to RIT. Distance to FPS, however, has no effect for the reason stated earlier. Household size, as expected, has a very large effect through higher demand for sugar despite a weakening effect of

TABLE **9.7e** Results of Tobit Estimation (Rajasthan—Sugar)

No. of Observations = 290 Prob>Chi-2 = 0.007
LR-chi2(13) = 29.03 Pseudo R2 = 0.036
Log Likelihood = −385.36
Rajasthan – SUGAR

	Coefficient			Marginal Effect
Land Owned	5.665	(1.94)	*	1.309
Square of Land Owned	−0.615	(−1.41)	–	−0.142
Land Gini	30.690	(1.96)	*	7.091
Proportion of BPL Cardholders in a Village	40.124	(3.28)	***	9.271
Ratio of PDS to Market Price (Sugar)	1,637.424	(2.2)	**	378.332
Price ratio (Sugar) – Squared	−1,128.157	(−2.15)	**	−260.665
Distance to FPS	−1.002	(−1.06)	–	−0.231
HH Size	−0.904	(−0.29)	–	−0.209
HH Size – Squared	0.015	(0.06)	–	0.003
No. of Adult Males	−0.558	(−0.27)	–	−0.129
No. of Adult Females	−1.462	(−0.58)	–	−0.338
Agricultural Wage Rate	0.063	(0.25)	–	0.015
Waiting time at FPS	0.005	(0.23)	–	0.001
Constant	−632.633	(−2.39)		
Sigma	*17.459*			
Left Censored Observations	*225*			
Uncensored Observations	*65*			

larger households. The longer the distance to a nearest town, the more supply constrained are the FPS and the lower are the real income gains.

Rajasthan

In the case of RIT through subsidized wheat, the effect of land owned—including that of its square—has a large positive effect on RIT, implying leakages to the better endowed on a very large scale. But there is a positive effect of the land Gini, implying that in villages with greater concentration of land distribution, real income gains were larger. As conjectured earlier and subject to verification, if there

TABLE 9.7f Results of Tobit Estimation (Maharashtra—Wheat)

No. of Observations = 483	Prob>Chi-2 = 0.000			
LR-chi2(12) = 51.13	Pseudo R2 = 0.015			
Log Likelihood = −1693.08				
Maharashtra – WHEAT				
	Coefficient			Marginal Effect
Land Owned	−2.442	(−1.03)	–	−0.970
Square of Land Owned	0.172	(1.61)	–	0.068
Land Gini	−106.369	(−2.45)	**	−42.243
Proportion of BPL Cardholders in a Village	201.499	(5.82)	***	80.023
Ratio of PDS to Market Price (Wheat)	2,096.669	(2.2)	**	832.668
Price Ratio (Wheat) – Squared	−2,652.538	(−2.28)	**	−1,053.425
Distance to FPS	−23.190	(−3.44)	***	−9.210
HH Size	21.402	(2.19)	**	8.500
HH Size – Squared	−1.758	(−1.97)	**	−0.698
No. of Adult Males	7.319	(1.17)	–	2.907
No. of Adult Females	−6.433	(−0.77)	–	−2.555
Agricultural Wage Rate	0.741	(1.6)	–	0.294
Constant	−533.245	(−2.8)		
Sigma	*92.055*			
Left Censored Observations	*230*			
Uncensored Observations	*253*			

is a large number of landless and near landless, manifesting in a higher Gini, their RIT may be higher. But this cannot be the entire explanation, as there are commodity-specific variations, as shown below. Also, this does not contradict the previous result which focuses on the positive effect of land ownership of individual households. Although fewer in number, such households may benefit more than the landless, but between villages, the higher proportion of landless in one may tilt real income gains in its favour. Distance to FPS has a negative effect. This is not surprising as FPS are not so well dispersed as in Andhra Pradesh. Nor does the agricultural wage rate at the village level have a significant effect. The hypothesized effect is positive as higher wage rates could result in higher demand for wheat. Somewhat surprisingly,

TABLE 9.7g Results of Tobit Estimation (Maharashtra—Rice)

No. of Observations = 483 Prob>Chi-2 = 0.000
LR-chi2(14) = 61.42 Pseudo R2 = 0.018
Maharashtra – RICE

	Coefficient			Marginal Effect
Land Owned	−2.491	(−1.08)	–	−0.968
Square of Land Owned	0.099	(0.94)	–	0.038
Land Gini	117.965	(2.64)	***	45.838
Proportion of BPL Cardholders in a Village	121.567	(3.23)	***	47.238
Ratio of PDS to Market Price (Wheat)	4,477.887	(2.72)	***	1,739.985
Price Ratio (Wheat) – Squared	−5,359.899	(−2.75)	***	−2,082.710
Ratio of PDS to Market Price (Rice)	−2,273.831	(−2.76)	***	−883.549
Price Ratio (Rice) Squared	2,209.008	(2.66)	***	858.360
Distance to FPS	0.227	(0.03)	–	0.088
HH Size	23.433	(2.46)	**	9.105
HH Size – Squared	−1.698	(−1.93)	*	−0.660
No. of Adult Males	1.856	(0.31)	–	0.721
No. of Adult Females	2.619	(0.32)	–	1.018
Agricultural Wage Rate	−0.469	(−0.96)	–	−0.182
Constant	−515.270	(−2.46)		
Sigma	*89.261*			
Left Censored Observations	*228*			
Uncensored Observations	*255*			

Source: (Tables 9.7a to 9.7g): Calculations based on primary data collected by R. Jha and R. Gaiha in 2007–8, from three Indian states, Rajasthan, Andhra Pradesh, and Maharashtra. Details available on request.

none of the demographic variables has a significant effect. In order to capture the effect of supply shortages, we experimented with proportion of BPL cardholders in village population. The presumption is that low margins could be offset by larger numbers of BPL cardholders.[14] This variable has the hypothesized positive effect on real incomes.

The results on subsidized rice are as follows. The effect of land owned is positive on RIT while that of its square is not significant. The land Gini does not influence real incomes. As in the case of wheat, we have considered both subsidized wheat and rice prices, and their squared values.

The combined effect of rice price subsidy (including its square) is negative, implying that the greater the rice price subsidy, the lower was the real income gain. This is not plausible. However, the combined effect of subsidized wheat price (including its squared value) is positive, implying that the higher the PDS wheat price ratio, the larger the demand for subsidized rice, and consequently, the higher is the RIT through subsidized rice. Distance has a weakly significant negative effect. None of the demographic variables has a significant effect on rice demand, and thus no real income effect. Controlling for all these effects, the higher the agricultural wage, the greater is the RIT. As in the case of wheat, the higher the proportion of BPL cardholders, the greater are the RIT through rice, implying, as argued earlier, more adequate supplies.

Results on RIT through subsidized sugar are somewhat uneven. Land owned is associated with a positive effect on RIT while that of its square is not significant. The land Gini has a large favourable effect on RIT. The combined effect of ratio of TPDS to market price and its square is negative and moderately large (in its absolute value). This implies that the larger the subsidy, the greater is the RIT, or vice versa. None of the demographic variables have a significant effect. Nor does agricultural wage rate at the village level have any effect. However, as a proxy for adequacy of supply, proportion of BPL cardholders in a village population have a large positive effect on real incomes.

Maharashtra

In the case of wheat, while land owned does not have a significant effect, its square has a significant positive effect. But the effect of the land Gini is negative and large (in absolute value), pointing to larger leakages to open markets. The ratio of TPDS to market price has a significant negative effect and the (absolute) value is large, implying that the larger the price subsidy, the greater was the RIT. But the longer the distance to FPS, the lower was the RIT.[15] The combined effect of household size and its square is positive. As argued earlier, on the assumption that the proportion of BPL cardholders is a proxy for supply adequacy, its effect on real income is positive and large.

There is no association between land owned (or its square), and RIT through subsidized rice. Somewhat surprisingly, the effect of the land Gini is reversed, compared with the effect on RIT through wheat. Instead of larger leakages, RIT through rice are substantially larger. Depending on whether the number of better endowed in terms of land are instrumental in not just larger leakages, but also more adequate supplies, this reversal of the wheat effect is not unlikely. Both ratios of TPDS to market price of wheat and rice (and their squares) have significant negative effects on RIT through subsidized rice. The (absolute) values of these effects are large. The larger the rice price subsidy, the greater is the RIT. A similar effect for wheat suggests complementarity between rice and wheat demand. As expected, household size has a significant positive effect on real income. As a proxy for adequacy of supply, the proportion of BPL cardholders has a large positive effect on RIT.

Thus, our analysis points to several factors—including demographic, land owned, land Gini, difference between TPDS and market prices, distance to FPS—determining RIT through subsidized wheat, rice, and sugar, and variation in these transfers across the three states.

UNIVERSAL FOOD SUBSIDY

In the context of dismal performance of the TPDS and desperation of the UPA government, the National Advisory Council (NAC) has enthusiastically endorsed a universal food subsidy under the aegis of a National Food Security Bill/Act (NFSB/NFSA).[16] In our view, this (as well as another extreme proposal to replace TPDS with a cash transfer system based on the biometric identity and multi-purpose smart cards)[17] are far from persuasive, if not escapist, as we believe that there is considerable scope for reform of the TPDS, and for better targeting of the poor with the existing outlay. Let us first examine why a universal food subsidy is unlikely to improve the public distribution of food.

There are strong advocates of a Right to Food (RTF) Act, given pervasive hunger and child malnutrition. Besides, there are legal compulsions. Article 21 (the fundamental 'right to life') of the Indian Constitution encompasses the RTF, while Article 47 of the Directive Principles directs the state to 'regard the raising of the level of nutrition and the standard of living of its people as among its primary duties'. Finally, the Supreme Court has issued several orders on fulfilment of food entitlements (Khera 2011).

Since RTF does not involve state provision of food, except under special circumstances of failures of duties to avoid and protect, during natural disasters, in an important sense it could be viewed as a right to policies (or, as 'a right to a right') that enables individuals to produce or acquire minimum food requirements (Osmani 2000). This may yield useful insights into whether non-fulfilment of the right to food is due to insufficiency of public resources, or due to policies followed, or both.

From this perspective, recent debates on the NFSB/NFSA have concentrated on a rigid interpretation of the RTF as being confined mostly to state provision of food.[18]

Our comments are anchored to a recent emphatic endorsement of the NAC proposal by Himanshu and Sen (2011). As elaborated below, their endorsement is contentious.

First, they insist that a universal PDS is the only option consistent with RTF, and, more contentiously, that feasible alternatives that are more universal and less targeted are more likely to be effective in benefiting the poor.[19] Second, between 1993–4 (a universal PDS) and 2004–5 (TPDS), the leakages grew enormously—from 19 per cent to 40 per cent (for rice); and from 41 per cent to 73 per cent (for wheat). Per capita per month consumption of TPDS rice and wheat remained unchanged, although TPDS off-take doubled and subsidy rose even more. There was, however, a slight improvement in access by the poorest 50 per cent of the population—from 28 per cent to 30 per cent. But this must be judged a colossal failure, given the massive cost of leakages. As noted earlier, the cost of transferring Re 1 to the poor is Rs 8.5. A considerable chunk of budgeted food subsidies (81 per cent in 2008–9) goes to the FCI, to cover its expenses for procurement, transportation, distribution, and for carrying over huge stocks. The high costs reflect inclusion errors, as well as corruption and leakages of grains, at all stages in the supply chain, from the procurement of grains by FCI to the final sales to eligible households (Svedberg 2012). Third, Himanshu and Sen (2011) are emphatic that the more universal the food subsidy—as in Tamil Nadu, among a few other states—the lower would be the leakage. There are two issues that are conflated in this proposition: first, the huge diversion of TPDS foodgrains to the market, and second, the losses during storage in open godowns. Whether a universal subsidy would reduce leakages to the market has little to do with how universal the food subsidy is, and more to do with the wedge between the market price and TPDS price, and trade margins for FPS. If procurements are higher, market price is likely to rise relative to the TPDS price, and market diversions would be larger.[20] As far as wastage is concerned, with larger procurements and inadequate storage facilities, wastage is also likely to be larger under a universal scheme. Fourth, a fraction of entitlements is bought by BPL households, thus limiting RIT to them. 30 per cent of total TPDS purchases of subsidized foodgrains (rice and wheat) are made by poor households with AAY or BPL ration cards.[21] Almost two-thirds of the poor (62.4 per cent), however, do not possess these cards, limiting their purchases to miniscule amounts. Add to this difficulty high transaction costs (long distances to FPS and waiting periods) and perceptions of poor quality and under-weighing to get a clearer picture of why the poor on average tend to buy amounts considerably lower than their entitlements (barely 15 kg of rice and wheat when the entitlement is 35 kg). As a result, the food subsidy per kg among poor households is slightly below Rs 4 in both rural and urban areas (Svedberg 2012). On the other hand, low margins to FPS act as a strong incentive to FPS to sell in the open market (Khera 2011).

Kumar and Ghosh (2012) estimate the cost of NFSB in the first three years, taking into account the costs of covering BPL and APL households in rural and urban areas, storage costs for the additional food procurement, leakages, provision of free nutritious meals during pregnancy and six months thereafter, and an additional maternity benefit of Rs 1000 per month, nutritional food to children—especially the malnourished—MDMS to those in lower and upper classes, and transportation costs to FPS works out to be a staggering Rs 500,000 crore.[22]

As an alternative, Svedberg (2012) and others are emphatic that the TPDS should be replaced with cash transfers (CT). A differentiated CT is proposed that includes three categories: (i) all SCs and STs, (ii) all casual labour households, and (iii) all households with no literate adult. Although proportions of poor are high in these categories, contrary to the assertion by Svedberg (2012), the inclusion errors are not small (even among casual labour households, 40 per cent are non-poor). CTs on a per person monthly basis range from Rs 33 for households meeting one criterion to Rs 100 for those who fulfil all three criteria. The total for the three sums up to Rs 472 billion, well within the 2010–11 budget of Rs 632 billion, leaving a balance of approximately Rs 160 billion for operation cost. While this is a meticulously worked out alternative, its optimism seems exaggerated for the following reasons that have plagued most anti-poverty interventions. Briefly, these include accurate targeting given the benefit of biometric identification under the Unique Identification (UID), which was nearly derailed and may take a few years to complete. Worse, the UID does not include socio-economic data that the three criteria require. In the absence of such data and the cash benefit being not-so-small per household, non-poor masquerading as acutely poor cannot be ruled out. Whether the operation cost would be fully covered by the amount proposed is far from evident. Finally, also admitted by Svedberg (2012), updating of the socio-economic database may not be feasible as frequently as required for accurate targeting. So this proposal is a *non-sequitur*.

A brief comment on the inclusion of the MDMS under the universal food subsidy is necessary as pesticide infected meals in Bihar resulted in tragic deaths of children, with other alarming accounts of how dreadful the meal quality has been in other parts of India and no remedial action.[23]

As Sinha (2013) observes, '.... loss of 23 innocent lives after consuming hot cooked meals in a school in Bihar has rightly shocked and angered people. The highly poisonous pesticide monocrotophos was found in children's food. This appears to be a case of poison in food rather than food poisoning'.

The MDMS is a decentralized programme, funded jointly by the central and state governments. While the food grain comes from FCI through the state food corporations, it is the School Management Committee (SMC) with the headmaster, Panchayati Raj Institutions (PRI) or other community representatives, and three-fourths representation of parents of children studying in that school that is given the responsibility to buy pulses, vegetables, oil, spices, firewood, and so on as conversion cost.

The MDM's favourable effects on school attendance and nutrition of poor children in government schools have been widely confirmed

(Afridi 2010; Khera 2013). Afridi (2010), for example, found positive nutrition effects among children in Madhya Pradesh—comparing nutrient intake on a school day with a non-school day—as nutrient intake of programme participants increased by 49 per cent to 100 per cent of the transfers; deficiency in protein reduced by 100 per cent, and iron deficiency by 10 per cent, all for a very small cost of 3 cents per child.

Even though SMCs and Mothers' Committees have been given key role of management, in practice a lot depends on the headmaster and the elected PRI representatives. Important questions are: how to strengthen the role of parents in the SMC, and, more broadly, how to make it a truly community-run programme as that is the best guarantee for quality food? Various proposals include: the headmaster, cook, and community representatives must mandatorily taste the food and certify its quality before it is consumed by children; clean water, sanitation (washing hands), and hygiene need to be systematically promoted; nutritionists, food regulators, and programme managers need to be inducted into the programme at all levels with proper health monitoring of the children; and food storage at the school level must receive greater attention with appropriate storage bins for all ingredients (Khera 2013; Sinha 2013). These proposals are overoptimistic, if not somewhat naïve, as for example, tasting of food by the headmistress of the school in Bihar where the tragedy occurred was mandatory, but not done despite protests by the cook and children themselves when 'black smoke' was observed and a foul smell was detected. The private contractors and bogus self-help groups come in for some stick in Khera (2013) as the dominant vested interests in MDM. Arguably, this is a somewhat exaggerated tirade as failure to regulate and monitor ought not to be overlooked. So while the proposals are long in description and of course merit serious consideration, they are short on their enforcement.

In brief, as in the case of the PDS, MDM needs a drastic overhaul.

TPDS, NREGS, AND NUTRITIONAL DEPRIVATION

Whether real income transfers through TPDS and NREGS mitigate undernutrition is analysed using primary date collected by Jha and Gaiha for 2007–8.[24] Some of the interesting findings of our analysis are reviewed here.

We first consider the nutritional profiles of Andhra Pradesh, Maharashtra, and Rajasthan, taking into account consumption of calories, proteins, and micronutrients—calcium, iron, carotene, thiamine, riboflavin, Vitamin C and niacin—(Jha *et al.* 2011). Using standard cut-off points for each, it turns out that not a single household in Andhra Pradesh was adequately nourished in all nine nutrients. Mean consumption of all nutrients except iron was below the respective cut-off point for nutritional adequacy. However, there was considerable inequality in nutrient consumption across the sample with the minimum cut-off for calories, for example, attained only by households in the top 10 per cent by calorie consumption.

The nutritional profile of Maharashtra is slightly better—1.3 per cent of the households were adequately nourished in all nutrients. As in Andhra Pradesh, there was considerable inequality in nutritional attainment with the minimum calorie norm reached only by the top 5 per cent of households for calorie consumption. In Rajasthan, barely 0.5 per cent of the households were adequately nourished across all nine nutrients. However, it had the lowest prevalence of deprivation across all nutrients (29 per cent of households). Only the top 12 per cent of households in calorie consumption crossed the minimum norm.

Our results point to varied effects of NREG and TPDS on the intake of various nutrients. Both NREG and PDS significantly increased the intake of calories, proteins, iron, among others, in these states. In the case of calcium, however, in Maharashtra, both PDS and NREG had positive and significant effects whereas neither was significant in Rajasthan. In Andhra Pradesh, on the other hand, only PDS had a significant effect on calcium consumption. These differences reflect the different ways in which the income from NREG and income transfer implicit in the PDS are spent, and the dietary preferences of households in these states.

Using participation measures in PDS and NREG, their effects on nutrient intake are compared in terms of their cost-effectiveness.[25] In Andhra Pradesh, in most cases, PDS had a larger effect than NREG. By contrast, in Maharashtra, NREG had larger effects in most cases. Rajasthan presents a more complex picture. For some nutrients (for example, calories, iron, and niacin), PDS had larger effects than NREG while for others (for example, protein, riboflavin), the latter had larger effects. So a general inference about the greater effectiveness of PDS or NREG is ruled out. Further, the effects of NREG wages on nutrient intake in many cases (for example, protein, calories, niacin) are larger than those of non-NREG income. This is not surprising as physically demanding tasks necessitate higher nutrient intake. This is, of course, not an issue in the context of RIT implicit in the PDS.

★★★

An important aspect of the assessment of the usefulness of any social welfare programme, particularly one that claims to be targeted towards the poor, is examining its incidence at the household level. This helps us directly understand whether the programme's benefits are reaching those for whom these were intended. Further, it becomes important to understand the factors determining household benefits from this programme. Such an analysis is particularly relevant for a social welfare programme such as the TPDS, given that the cost associated with it is spiralling uncontrollably.

This chapter used primary data from a representative sample of rural households collected from three Indian states—Rajasthan, Andhra Pradesh, and Maharashtra—to understand various access issues related to the TPDS. It documents the fact that the programme is not well targeted in some instances, that both the poor and non-poor get subsidized by the TPDS, and that the distribution of benefits by caste, waiting time for buying food through FPS, and land ownership categories are not what was intended. We also analysed the extent to which RIT from wheat, rice, and sugar under TPDS are determined by a household's economic status, its demographic characteristics, price subsidy (at the village level), transaction costs of buying from FPS, and supply constraints.

Our analysis corroborates the influence of these factors. Land as a proximate indicator of economic status has mixed effects varying by commodity and state. Specifically, there are a few cases where land owned and RIT are lower (rice in Andhra Pradesh, and wheat and rice in Maharashtra), suggesting that those not so well endowed (and by implication BPL households) benefited more. Inequality in land distribution takes different forms (concentrations of landless and near landless, or of the well-endowed) and influences real incomes in complex ways (leakages and larger supply or just leakages). As a result, the effects vary by commodity and state (negative for rice in Andhra Pradesh, and positive for wheat in Rajasthan and rice in Maharashtra). The extent of price subsidy, in most cases, results in larger RIT. Household size influences positively demand and real incomes in some cases (rice and sugar in Andhra Pradesh, and wheat in Maharashtra) and negatively in other cases (wheat and rice in Rajasthan), depending on whether economies of scale in food expenditure matter more. There is some evidence of transaction cost (for example, distance to FPS) limiting income gains (wheat in Rajasthan and Maharashtra). There is overwhelming support for supply inadequacy limiting income gains, given proximate indicators.

Our analysis shows that careful attention must be given to reducing transaction costs—long distances to be travelled, long queues and waiting periods, and under-weighing by FPS. A better network of FPS, higher margins and adequate supplies would go a long way in making the TPDS more cost-effective. A real culprit is the FCI with its abysmal inefficiency in procuring, storing, and distributing food. Above all, top priorities include livelihood expansion opportunities in rural areas, and food price stabilization—two areas in which UPA's track record has, and continues to be, unimpressive.

If, instead, a revamped TPDS on a much smaller scale is combined with more sensible policies that aim to augment productivity in agriculture, avoid market imperfections that come in the way of remunerative farm gate food prices, and expand livelihood options, fulfilment of food entitlements may be far less costly.

So, even with existing budget outlays, there is considerable scope for better targeting the poor, enhancing their food entitlements, and improving their nutritional status.

ANNEXURE

TABLE 9A.1 Definitions of Variables Used in the Tobit Analysis

Variables	Definition
Dependent Variable	
Real Income Transfer from PDS	Real income transfer through PDS is computed separately for each of the three food commodities by multiplying the (Market price – PDS price) by the quantity of food item bought by the household

(continued)

TABLE 9A.1 Continued

Variables	Definition
Explanatory Variables	
Land Owned	Land Owned by Household in acres
Square of Land Owned	Square of Land Owned by Household in acre
Land Gini	Gini Coefficient of land distribution at the village level
Proportion of BPL card-holders in a Village	Proportion of BPL card holders in Village
Ratio of PDS to Market Price (Wheat)	(PDS Price/Market price) for wheat at Village level
Price Ratio (Wheat) – Squared	Square of Ratio of Village Level PDS to Market price – Wheat
Ratio of PDS to Market Price (Rice)	(PDS Price/Market price) for rice at Village level
Price Ratio (Rice) Squared	Square of Ratio of Village Level PDS to Market price – Rice
Ratio of PDS to Market Price (Sugar)	(PDS Price/Market price) for sugar at Village level
Price ratio (Sugar) – Squared	Square of Ratio of Village Level PDS to Market price – Sugar
Distance to FPS	Distance from village to the nearest FPS in km.
HH Size	Household Size – number of members in the household
HH Size – Squared	Square of Household Size
No. of Adult Males	Number of Adult Males in the Household
No. of Adult Females	Number of Adult Females in the Household
Agricultural Wage Rate	Village level Wage Rate for casual Agricultural Labourer (Rs per day)
Distance to Nearest Town	Distance from village to nearest town in km.
Distance to Nearest Town – Squared	Square of Distance from village to nearest Town in km.
Waiting Time at FPS	Total Time spent in buying Foodgrains from FPS per month (hours)

Source: Calculations based on primary data collected by R. Jha and R. Gaiha in 2007–8, from three Indian states, Rajasthan, Andhra Pradesh, and Maharashtra. Details available on request.

Note: For rural areas, PSU is a village, and, for urban areas, it is a town.

NOTES

1. Food subsidy is defined as the excess of market price of a commodity and the subsidized prices multiplied by the amount sold through the PDS.

2. This scheme was launched in 2000 to help 10 million of the poor population (or 2 million households) who could not afford two square meals a day. Given this measure, and generally low estimates of the poorest characterized in this way, the targeting has been uneven and unsatisfactory across states.

3. Himanshu and Sen (2011) provide a recent, emphatic endorsement of this view; for a critique, see Gaiha *et al.* (2012b).

4. Government regulates FPS owners by stipulating the maximum amount they can sell and the profit margin. Hence, their profits depend on the number of customers.

5. The amount varies between rural and urban poor, but slightly (Svedberg 2012).

6. Details will be furnished on request.

7. Marginal effects are also computed on the conditional expectation $E(y \mid y>0, \mathbf{x})$. For details, see Greene (2003).

8. The Gini coefficient is often used to measure inequality in income distribution or any other distribution (for example, land ownership). It ranges from 0 (perfect equality when all individuals have the same income) to 1 (maximum inequality when 1 person has the entire income). As Sen (1997) shows, the sensitivity of this measure depends not on the size of the income levels, but on the number of people in between them. Specifically, the Gini coefficient implies a welfare function which is just a weighted sum of different people's income levels with the weights being determined by the rank order—order of the position of the person in the ranking by income level. He constructs an example to demonstrate how the weights on the income transfer to the richer person increase when the number of people in a given income gap (between the not-so-rich and the richer person) increases without any change in incomes of the two individuals (Sen 1997, pp. 32–3). The important point, therefore, is that rank order weights could change with numbers between two incomes changing, and consequently the Gini coefficient.

9. For definitions of acute and moderately poor, and moderately non-poor and relatively affluent, see Table 9.6.

10. For kerosene, out of the villages for which we have data, 8 villages are in Rajasthan, 19 villages in Andhra Pradesh and 7 villages in Maharashtra. However, given the measure of participation in TPDS, no further comments are made.

11. See, for example, Atkinson (1987).

12. The actual poverty cut-off point is Rs 450 (per capita per month).

13. Note that in this section, 'participating households' are those households which bought food such as wheat, rice or sugar from TPDS during 2007.

14. Recall that Kochar (2005) relies on the number of APL households. We did not use this as the numbers of APL households in our samples were small.

15. Note that while the mean distance to FPS is lowest in Maharashtra, its standard deviation is higher than in Andhra Pradesh.

16. The original proposal has undergone changes and is awaiting passage in the current monsoon session of Parliament. For a detailed comment on the earlier proposal, see Gaiha *et al.* (2012b).

17. It is far from evident how the economic status of a household will be determined through a biometric identification without accurate assessment of household assets. Land records, for example, continue to be fudged on a large scale and incomes are hard to define and measure among the self-employed in agriculture in rural areas.

18. National Food Security Act implies ratification of NFSB by parliament. As the debate continues unabated and the Bill's passage without major modifications is not unlikely, we prefer NFSB to NFSA.

19. This is mistaken as a right to food could be interpreted as a right to a right, or, more specifically, as a right to sensible livelihood expansion and food price stabilization policies (Gaiha 2003).

20. As pointed out by Svedberg (2012), the demand for foodgrains in the Himanshu and Sen proposal (2011) is between 60–100 million tonnes per year. The upper-end estimates correspond to about half the annual rice and wheat production, and is equal to all grains that are marketed. But surprisingly, they (and other proponents of a universal food subsidy), do not foresee serious market disruption from such state monopsony, an issue that has cropped up prominently in recent debates on the NFSB. For a related analysis, see Gaiha *et al.* (2007).

21. Under the AAY scheme, the poorest of the poor, subject to difficulties of identification, are given the option to buy food at even more subsidized prices than BPL households. Note that some of these estimates differ from those reported by Svedberg (2012).

22. Himanshu and Sen (2011) refrain from giving an estimate of the total budget requirements for their proposed expansion of the TPDS. However, even if the pure subsidy component increases from 31 per cent in 2004–5 to 50 per cent, the total fiscal burden would be twice their estimated Rs 794 billion, or close to Rs 1600 billion. This would increase the total costs of the programme from about 1 per cent of NNP at present to 2 per cent (Svedberg 2012).

23. Similar issues have arisen in Delhi where centralized kitchens supply unhygienic and unsafe meals, but parents, children, even teachers do not really

know where to complain. Samples regularly fail quality tests, but not much has happened to remedy this (Khera 2013).

24. These are obtained by estimating an equation in which the dependent variable is nutrient intake (including micronutrients) and the explanatory variables comprise TPDS participation and NREG wage, non-wage income (all three appropriately instrumented) and other household characteristics. To compare the effect of a change in TPDS participation with that of a change in NREG wage on nutrient intake, we use one standard deviation increase in these variables. For details, see Jha *et al.* (2011).

25. The effects on nutrient intake are contingent upon a modest real income transfer (Rs 100 per month or a day's NREG wage). For details, see Jha *et al.* (2011).

10 Policies, Implementation, and Impact

Raghav Gaiha, Raghbendra Jha,
and Vani S. Kulkarni

The main findings are reviewed from a policy perspective that draws upon extant evidence from India and elsewhere. The vision that we construct is necessarily incomplete, but illuminates successes and failures in designing policies and in their implementation, and delineates priorities.

THE NUTRITION PUZZLE

Recent evidence points to a puzzle. Despite rising incomes, there has been sustained decline in per capita nutrient intake. In an important contribution, Deaton and Dréze (2009) offer an analysis of the decline in nutrient intake over the period 1983 to 2004. Their principal findings are that the average calorie consumption was about 10 per cent lower in rural areas in 2004–5 than in 1983. The proportionate decline was larger among the more affluent sections of the population, and negligible for the population in the bottom quartile of the per capita expenditure scale. In urban areas, there was a slight change in average calorie intake over this period. Proteins also experienced a drop in per capita consumption, whereas the intake of fat increased in both rural and urban areas. As incomes rose over this period, these declines are puzzling.

Deaton and Dréze are emphatic that the declines are not attributable to changes in relative prices as an aggregate measure of the price of food—treated synonymous with the price of calories—changed little during this period. So the puzzle boils down to this: per capita calorie consumption is lower at every given level of per capita household expenditure, across the expenditure scale, at low levels of per capita expenditure as well as high; that is, there is a steady downward shift of the calorie Engel curve.[1]

Instead, they attribute the downward shift of the calorie Engel curve to lower calorie 'requirements', associated mainly with better health and lower activity levels. Specifically, they draw attention to major expansions in availability of safe drinking water, vaccination rates, transport facilities, and ownership of various effort-saving durables.

We offer a different explanation of changes in the consumption of calories, protein, and fats over the more recent period, 1993–2004. Our results show consistently robust food price and expenditure effects. Besides, shifts in food price elasticities over time are significant, indicating changes in price responsiveness of demand. Over and above these effects, there are shifts in demands due to factors other than those specified in the demand equations. In the context of calories, for example, it is plausible that part of the reduction in their consumption was due to health improvements and less strenuous activity levels. So, while the Deaton and Dréze (2009) explanation is not rejected, it is arguable that it is complementary to the demand-based explanations.

DIET DIVERSIFICATION

A key feature of the economic and demographic transition is the change in the nature of the Indian diet, driven by expansion of the middle class, urbanization, higher female participation in labour force, emergence of nuclear two-income families, a sharp age divide in food preferences (with younger age-groups more susceptible to new foods advertised in the media), rapid growth of supermarkets and fast food outlets. Dietary changes are characterized by a substitution of traditional staples by milk/ghee/butter, meat/fish/poultry, fruits and vegetables, eggs, and vanaspati oil. As these are linked to intake of calories, proteins, and fats with varying importance, we examined whether diet diversification could explain lower calorie intake over the period 1993–2004.

While the food diversity index (FDI) is itself influenced by food prices, affluence, size of the middle class, urbanization, the former in turn is linked to calorie intake after accounting for the influence of food prices, expenditure, and various household characteristics and their location. Specifically, the greater the food diversity, the lower was the calorie intake. Although this link has been hinted at or simply glossed over in recent studies, this is the first robust confirmation.

Eating out contributes to diet diversification. It refers to meals or snacks served in restaurants, roadside eating places, tea and snack shops, and street vendors. Eating out is pervasive, going by the fact that about 30 per cent of the households did so. It is a feature of not just the metros or urban areas, but also of urban slums and rural areas, though it is less pervasive in the last two areas. Eating out was not just more pervasive among the metro residents, but they also spent larger amounts. Other factors that contributed to larger spending on eating out include number of adult males and females in paid employment, share of business income in household income, and (relative) affluence of a household. As the mix of food served includes fast food (for example, burgers, pizzas, *pakoras*, *samosas*), junk food (chips, chocolate, soft drinks), instant foods (noodles, soup powder), and street foods (*chaat*, *tikki*, *golgappa*), they are high in sugar, saturated fat, salt, and calorie content which are associated with higher risks of obesity, hypertension, and impaired glucose tolerance.[2] A related concern is that some of these foods are prepared, handled, and stored in unhygienic conditions that lead to microbiological contamination.

A major worry is exposure of school children and adolescents to these foods. They are lured by convincing marketing strategies through the media and peer pressure. Consumption of diet high in sugar, saturated fat, and calories in childhood can lead to early development of obesity and cardiovascular diseases.

CALORIE THRESHOLD AS NUTRITION NORM

If the proportions of undernourished are measured using fixed calorie norms, there is an increase in the prevalence of undernutrition (synonymous with calorie-deprivation). Even if the calorie norms are taken to be lower, a grim picture emerges. Using fixed calorie norms to measure undernutrition is suspect due to familiar reasons. So we considered an alternative measure that relies on consumption behaviour, as opposed to calorie norms. The basic argument is that individuals tend to switch away from the cheapest source of calories (staple food), after surpassing subsistence, towards more expensive sources of calories. If this switch occurs at a certain share of calories from staples, all those above the threshold are counted as undernourished (Jensen and Miller 2011).

Our analysis with the National Sample Survey data for 1993 and 2004 shows that such a measure is potentially misleading as it confines variation in the calorie share to a measure of wealth, ignoring the role of relative prices. Besides, the estimates of undernourished are vitiated by the failure to distinguish between those who are above the calorie threshold at extremely low expenditures and those with much higher expenditures. As these changed differently over the period 1993–2004, and, arguably, call for different policies, the new measure has limited analytical and policy appeal. Indeed, the neglect of food price stabilization in mitigating undernutrition is worrying.

So, research must focus on a more appropriate range of calorie and other nutrient requirements that better reflect evolving lifestyles that are more sedentary, less strenuous activity patterns, and improvements in social epidemiology of infectious diseases. Notional adjustments will not do as their bases are uncertain.

WHY DO POVERTY NUTRITION TRAPS (PNTs) MATTER?

Income shocks are frequent and often pervasive. Although India has graduated to an emerging economy with high rates of growth in recent years, these continue to be volatile. Domestic factors include monsoon failures that affect not just agricultural growth, but also overall growth. Monsoon failures often raise the spectre of a drought, rising food prices, and large-scale impoverishment. Besides, the continuing Eurozone crisis on the heels of the global financial crisis and recession hurt the Indian economy.[3] The deceleration of the GDP growth rate in the first quarter and further deceleration in the next manifest the vulnerability of the Indian economy to such shocks. The PNT are of considerable significance in this context. Our analysis demonstrated the large pool of undernourished and higher prevalence in recent years despite lack of a consensus on nutritional norms. As income shocks are likely to make it harder for the undernourished to participate in the labour market and to earn lower wages, the PNT will persist. In other words, the undernourished are less likely to break this trap. Our analysis confirmed this. In particular, female workers are more prone to PNT than male workers, and there is persistent gender inequality in rural India. As a result, the focus shifts to lack of nutritional adequacy as a precondition for participation in labour market activities. So, while income remains important in improving nutritional status of both adults and children, under certain conditions, the interdependence between the two cannot be overlooked. If our analysis is valid, nutritional supplements are also important in enhancing labour market prospects in an agrarian economy with efficiency wages. Although programmes such as NREG supplement incomes and increase nutrients' intake, an analysis suggests that the benefits to those better endowed in terms of BMI are greater.

IS PERSISTENCE OF CHILD UNDERNUTRITION REMEDIABLE?

More than 6,000 children under five years die every day in India due to malnourishment or lack of basic micronutrients such as vitamin A, iron, iodine, zinc, or folic acid. This is hardly surprising as India is one of a few countries with the worst levels of low birth weight, underweight, and stunting among children in BRIC and SAARC countries.

As the reduction of malnutrition levels has been slow, the prevalence rates are high enough to cause concern, especially since they persist amidst a phase of impressive economic growth.[4] The high levels of child malnutrition potentially impact a country's prospects for continued economic growth as child malnutrition in early years may result in malnutrition and lower cognitive skills in adult years. Additionally, it is a humanitarian concern requiring policy makers and international communities to refocus their policy priorities on direct and indirect interventions to reduce children's malnutrition.

Although children are one-third of India's billion plus population, their share in the Union budget is under 5 per cent, of which 70 per cent is allocated for education, and barely 11 per cent for health. So the funds allocated for child health are a small fraction of the funds allocated (Mendelson and Chaudhuri 2009).

Our analysis, based on a composite indicator of anthropometric failure (CIAF) of children, that allows for simultaneous anthropometric failures (for example, underweight, stunting, and wasting) among children under five years, reveals a grimmer story of child undernutrition than conventional indicators do. The CIAF is more pervasive than conventional indicators of underweight, stunted, or wasted children. The former is about 59 per cent. Among the subcategories, stunting and underweight, and stunting alone account for well over half of the CIAF. For policy purposes, it is useful to know the total burden of malnutrition so that appropriate budgetary allocations are made for child development.

The disaggregated classification of anthropometric failures points to greater susceptibility to infectious diseases such as diarrhoea and acute respiratory infection (ARI). The prevalence of diarrhoea was highest among those children who were simultaneously stunted and underweight, followed by those who were wasted, underweight, and stunted relative to no failure. The prevalence of ARI was highest too among stunted and underweight children.

Noting that the results vary with the nutrition indicators used and the period(s) covered, a distillation of determinants of CIAF and conventional indicators of child malnutrition is given below.[5]

Maternal education reduces child undernutrition, as it is linked to better child care and healthier diets. Mother's age also reduces child undernutrition. Women's empowerment captured through difference in male–female earnings further reduces it. An alternative indicator of women's empowerment, ratio of mother's education to father's, has a similar effect, implying greater bargaining power of women in allocating more resources for children, and preparation and composition of food. Income/wealth reduces child nutrition, but there are other factors unrelated to income that are just as important as income, if not more. In the context of stunting, for example, income has a weaker role in reducing it than, say, easier access to drinking water, and sanitation and hygiene facilities. The number of stunted children is positively related to the number of children under five years in a household, presumably because of a birth order effect.

Scheduled Castes (SCs) and Scheduled Tribes (STs)—the two most disadvantaged groups—recorded much higher rates of child malnutrition.

Food prices affect child malnutrition significantly as changes in relative prices induce substitution between food commodities and in nutrient intake. In a few cases, the food price effects are larger than those of income/wealth.[6]

As child malnutrition is a form of 'hidden' hunger, the potential for reduction through greater media exposure should not be overlooked.

In what follows, we will address two major concerns: one is the imperative of women's empowerment, and the second is inconsistencies between Integrated Child Development Services (ICDS) and National Rural Health Mission (NRHM).

Women's Empowerment

Of particular importance is women's autonomy in fertility decisions and allocation of household resources. Early marriages result in frequent pregnancies, low birth weight babies, lesser attention to them, and greater stunting.

Let us first consider key links between mother's health and child nutrition. Undernutrition begins in the utero: a malnourished mother is likely to give birth to a baby of low birth weight—the single most important predictor of child survival. According to NFHS-3, close to a third of Indian women suffer from chronic energy deficiency and have a BMI of less than 18.5.[7]

A second link is through breastfeeding and complementary feeding. The status is dismal. According to NFHS-3, the initiation of breastfeeding within an hour of birth was 24.5 per cent. Worse, complementary feeding along with continued breastfeeding in 6–9 months is 55.8 per cent. With this adverse start in life, undoing the damage is difficult. Education in the importance of breastfeeding and complementary feeding is crucial for lowering child undernutrition (Gupta *et al.* 2010; Mendelson and Chaudhuri 2009).

A woman's control over resources within the household affects her children.[8] Evidence supports the view that income or assets controlled by women are more likely to be spent on items that benefit children and themselves, such as food, clothing, and health care, than assets controlled by men. A revealing statistic from NFHS-3 is that malnutrition among children below three years born to illiterate mothers (55 per cent) is more than twice the level (26 per cent) among mothers with more than 10 years of education. What this statistic points to is that both child malnutrition and education are strongly correlated with women's social status (Mendelson and Chaudhuri 2009; Ruel *et al.* 2013; Smith *et al.* 2003).

But if the empowerment argument is valid, it is not just education of women, but also whether it is high relative to that of men that deserves emphasis, as also their earnings relative to those of men. So expansion of female education and employment opportunities would not just enhance women's autonomy and social status, but also lead to better child nutrition.

An extreme form of lack of women's autonomy is reflected in domestic violence against them. An important contribution (Ackerson and Subramanian 2008) sheds light on how such violence aggravates malnutrition among them and their children. The associations between domestic violence and various nutritional outcomes were in the same direction and of the same approximate strength for children as they were for women. In other words, domestic violence aggravated malnutrition among both women and children.[9]

Public policy interventions that enhance women's educational attainments and employment options, and modify inheritance laws in their favour will make a huge difference.[10]

Effectiveness of ICDS?

Two major nationwide public interventions are Integrated Child Development Services (ICDS), and National Rural Health Mission (NRHM). Our focus here is on the inconsistency between them.

ICDS targets long-term nutrition and development of children. It provides nutritional supplements, vaccinations, health check-ups and referral services, and day care.

NRHM is another health programme for improving health care delivery across rural India. The mission, initially mooted for seven years (2005–12), proposes a number of new mechanisms for health care delivery, including training local residents as 'Accredited Social Health Activists' (ASHA), and the *Janani Surakshay Yojana* (motherhood protection programme). It also aims at improving hygiene and sanitation infrastructure.

ICDS has an unimpressive track record. A World Bank review (2005) found a few successes, but little impact on child malnutrition.[11] It recommended a larger share of public investment towards younger children (0–3 years), and most vulnerable in states with the highest malnutrition, and a shift of emphasis from food delivery to changing family-based feeding and caring behaviour.

Attention has been drawn to operational inconsistencies between ICDS and NRHM in the identification of children suffering from severe acute malnutrition (SAM) (Prasad *et al.* 2012). NFHS-3 data show that about eight million children suffer from SAM.

The ICDS, through the *anganwadi* centres and *anganwadi* workers (AWWs), monitors growth of children under six years, identifies children who are malnourished, and provides follow up care (including referrals). In states/districts with a Nutrition Rehabilitation Centre (NRC) under NRHM, the AWW refers children who are severely underweight to the NRC. As a large number of cases referred by AWW do not fit the SAM criteria (58–75 per cent), they are sent back. Those admitted for treatment are usually discharged after fourteen days. In the absence of community-based management of malnutrition, this practice compromises the investment made during the fourteen days.

A community-based programme for management of SAM children could be led by the ICDS, since an anganwadi centre exists in every village. The AWW could be trained to identify children who are SAM, and screen children for referral to NRCs. A combination of therapeutic food, nutrition counselling, regular monitoring, and community mobilization could be adopted to substantially reduce child malnutrition.

In brief, the task is challenging, but there are grounds for optimism.

IS THERE A CASE FOR A UNIVERSAL FOOD SUBSIDY?

Our analysis of three states (Andhra Pradesh, Maharashtra, and Rajasthan) shows variation in real income transfers (RIT) through Targeted Public Distribution System (TPDS). Mean RIT was lowest among acutely poor households in Rajasthan; it was higher among the poor than among the moderately non-poor and (relatively) affluent; and it was highest among the (relatively) affluent in Maharashtra.

RIT vary for various reasons, but three are emphasized here: (i) the larger the food price subsidy (or the difference between the market price and TPDS price) in most cases, the larger is the RIT; (ii) transaction costs (for example, distance to FPS, waiting time in queues) limit income transfers; and (iii) there is robust support for supply inadequacy limiting income gains, largely due to diversions driven by measly margins offered to FPS.

Comparison of nutritional effects of NREGS and TPDS offers an interesting contrast. NREGS wage and TPDS participation significantly increase the intake of protein, carbohydrates, calories, phosphorous, iron, thiamine, and niacin in Andhra Pradesh, Maharashtra, and Rajasthan. In Andhra Pradesh, in most cases, TPDS had a larger effect than NREGS. By contrast, in Maharashtra, NREG had larger effects in most cases. Rajasthan presents a more complex picture. For some nutrients (for example, calories, iron, and niacin), TPDS has larger effects than NREG while for others (for example, protein, riboflavin) the latter has larger effects. So a general inference about the greater effectiveness of TPDS or NREG is ruled out. Further, the effects of NREG wages on nutrient intake in many cases (for example, protein, calories, niacin) are larger than those of non-NREG income. This is not surprising as physically demanding tasks necessitate higher nutrient intake.

Recent debates on the National Food Security Bill (NFSB) have concentrated on a rigid interpretation of the right to food (RTF) as being confined mostly to state provision of food. Indeed, it has been argued that in an important sense the RTF is a right to a right, or a right to sensible livelihood and food price policies that enable individuals to produce or acquire minimum food requirements. Except under emergencies, the assertion that a universal food subsidy is the only option consistent with the RTF is mistaken.

Although the procurement amounts estimated in different versions of a universal food subsidy vary, some important facts and difficulties are overlooked.

- In recent years, the leakages have grown enormously. Per capita per month consumption of PDS rice and wheat remained unchanged, although PDS off-take doubled and subsidy rose even more. There was, however, a slight improvement in access by the poorest 50 per cent of the population. But this must be judged a colossal failure, given the massive cost of leakages.

- Whether a universal subsidy would reduce these leakages substantially is contentious. Often two distinct issues are conflated. One is the huge diversion to the market, and the other is the losses during storage in open godowns. Whether a universal subsidy would reduce diversion to market has little to do with how universal the subsidy is, and more to do with low margins of FPS and the wedge between the market and PDS price. With larger procurements and given storage capacity, wastage is likely to be greater.
- The logistics of procurement are formidable. Even if we go by the arguably low foodgrain requirements of 60 million tonnes under the universal scheme, contested by many, a question is whether such a massive exercise of procurement and distribution can be handled by a centralized agency such as the Food Corporation of India (FCI).[12] In 2002–4, it cost Rs 134 per quintal to procure wheat, but the cost of moving the same quintal was over Rs 289. It is far from self-evident that the government should incur such massive expenditure for moving foodgrains to and fro in a centralized system that operates. The initiative to outsource some of the logistical work to private grain traders in recent years is sensible, but the scale and magnitude of procurement envisaged under the NFSB could easily become unmanageable.

If, instead, a revamped PDS on a much smaller scale is combined with more sensible policies that aim to augment low productivity in agriculture, avoid market imperfections that come in the way of remunerative farm gate food prices, and expand livelihood options, fulfilment of food entitlements may be far less costly. The long and short of it is that the PDS cries out for reforms without which more ambitious interventions are just as likely to fail.

Is unconditional cash transfer (CT) an option? In our view, it is not. A specific proposal of differentiated CT is a *non-sequitur*. There is a strong presumption of accurate targeting, given the benefit of biometric identification under the Unique Identification (UID), which was nearly derailed and may take a few years to complete. As UID does not include socio-economic data that will minimize the inclusion error under the three criteria, accurate targeting is a mere assertion.

So, even with the existing outlay, the benefits to the poor may be much larger in a drastically overhauled TPDS.

A related concern is gross mismanagement of the Mid-Day Meal Scheme (MDMS) with tragic deaths of twenty-three school children in a school in Bihar in July 2013. Less tragic but alarming reports of unhygienic and unsafe meals served in other states (for example, Delhi) with no remedial action also abound. Although the MDMS has had favourable effects on school attendance of children from the poor sections, and their nutrition, little attention has been given to monitoring the quality of meals served. Homilies are spewed out on strengthening of School Management Committees (SMC) comprising headmaster, Panchayati Raj Institutions (PRI), or other community representatives, and three-fourths representation of parents of children studying in that school, but concrete action plans remain neglected in the hope that drastic overhaul would somehow come about. Thus passionate pleas to incorporate it in the new NFSB are just that, and lack merit.

HEALTH RISKS

Dietary transition involves not just a more varied and nutritionally balanced diet and higher levels of food hygiene, but also consumption of energy-dense foods—high in salts, fats, and sugars—especially through fast foods that are linked to higher prevalence of diet-related non-communicable diseases (NCDs).

The excess energy from these foods may affect children and adults within the same household differently. Children may use up the excess energy and still remain underweight while adults are more likely to gain weight. Intra-household food allocation biases between adults and children, on the one hand, and between males and females, on the other, compound these effects.

About 62 per cent of the total disease burden (including injuries) is now attributable to NCDs, a larger share than communicable diseases and maternal and child health (MCH) issues. But communicable diseases (for example, tuberculosis, respiratory infections, and water and vector-borne disease) are still prominent in the total population, reflecting a 'double disease burden'.

Although India lags behind other developing countries in the epidemiological transition—decline in infectious disease mortality compensated for increasingly by higher mortality from chronic degenerative NCDs—there is some evidence of this transition taking place.

The estimated deaths from NCDs are projected to rise from 3.78 million in 1990 (40.46 per cent of all deaths) to 7.63 million in 2020 (66.70 per cent of all deaths).

As the demographic transition advances, and the population ages without associated improvements in living conditions, nutrition, and better access to health services, it is not surprising that ageing is a key factor in the growing burden of NCDs. Affluence also has a significant role through lifestyle changes and dietary composition. As caste affiliation better captures aspects of non-monetary deprivation, those at the bottom of the caste hierarchy (STs) have much lower prevalence of these diseases. Somewhat surprising is the low effect of overweight/obesity on NCDs.

The shift of the disease burden toward NCDs will increase demand on the health care system. With more health care currently financed with private out-of-pocket resources, it will be increasingly harder for households to escape poverty while more will be driven into poverty. As rural population migrates to urban areas, the associated lifestyle changes are likely to elevate NCD risks. Extreme poverty and foetal and early childhood undernutrition are likely to create a large pool of those at elevated risk.

The policy challenge is how to address the 'double disease' burden, and, in particular, the spectre of rising disabilities and deaths due to NCDs.

HEALTHY FOOD CHOICES?

The interplay between (relative) food prices and individual food choices poses difficult policy questions. The first question is whether (relative) food prices could be altered.

Diets rich in legumes, other vegetables, and coarse grains are disappearing as a result of major global developments in technology, liberalization of trade, marketing, and mass media. For example, new techniques were developed for cheaply removing oils from oilseeds. Breeding techniques to increase the oil content of these seeds accompanied the processing shifts, and higher income countries saw a large increase in the availability of cheap vegetable oils. By 2010, inexpensive oils were available throughout the developing world. Another example is the beginning of a livestock revolution in the developing world, resulting in substantial increases in the production of dairy products, eggs, and poultry. A key component of food system changes is modern food distribution and sales. There has been a rapid penetration of supermarkets that are either part of multinational or domestic chains. As a result, access to cheaper, processed foods that are high in fat, added sugar, and salt increased. Liberalization of food trade under WTO further facilitated this access.

So a large shift occurred in (relative) food prices in favour of animal-source foods, edible oils, and other key global commodities (Popkin *et al.* 2012). Given these global forces, domestic, monetary, and fiscal policies have a limited role in altering (relative) prices. As monetary policies are more effective in influencing the general price level, our comments are confined to aspects of fiscal policy (for example, subsidies and taxes) and regulation.

Our evidence suggests that both income supplementation (through, for example, NREGS) and food subsidy through PDS help improve intake of calories, proteins, and micronutrients. The costs, however, have escalated and without a drastic overhaul of these programmes, the fiscal burden is likely to be unsustainable.

Taxation of selected food items and beverages—especially sugar-sweetened beverages—is an option. Mexico is a case in point in how to reduce sugar-sweetened beverage consumption in schools, and thereby reduce calories consumed from beverages. About twenty countries have banned all sugary beverages from schools and twelve have banned 100 per cent fruit juices as well. While banning is a drastic step, available evidence points to potential benefits of taxation of sugary beverages, tobacco, alcohol, and fast foods.[13]

Whether voluntary initiatives on the part of global and national companies make a difference is unclear. First, there is no clear evidence that voluntary pledges by global companies will be linked to reduced energy intake, improved diet quality, or reduced obesity. Moreover, such pledges are mostly focused on USA, Europe, or other high income countries, and not the low-and middle-income countries. Even if these companies do reduce marketing the calorie content of their products, it is not unlikely that these products would simply be replaced by those of local companies.[14]

Current food policies/programmes in India—the ICDS (for children <6 years), the MDMS (for school children), and the TPDS—are focused on reducing hunger and malnutrition to the neglect of higher-quality foods (Dréze and Goyal 2003; Ramachandran 2010).[15] This runs the risk of increased weight gain and obesity.

The role of mass media—TVs, newspapers, films—has expanded considerably in recent years. The global penetration is such that hardly any household, village, or urban centre is missed. Children and adults are 'assaulted with visions of eating and drinking that are creating global shifts in food demand. Thus, a prime target for combating obesity is media control, though all initiatives ... have focused only on marketing to children and not on the total marketing environment' (Popkin *et al.* 2012: 16).

In India, media advertisement and publicity are under the overall authority of Ministry of Information and Broadcasting, Government of India. A committee has been constituted to review the complaints, decide whether the advertisement violates the rules, and issue a notice to TV channels in case of violation. But guidelines related to food quality are still not formulated (FSSAI 2012). Despite claims to the contrary, effective implementation of food safety standards has a long way to go.

Food and nutrition labelling is fast becoming a global initiative, with emphasis on 'nutrition facts' panels on foods, but also on developing systems for identifying which foods and beverages are deemed healthy according to the customs of each country.[16] This is a promising initiative as the global food supply increases in complexity, and consumers increasingly shift consumption to processed and packaged foods, and shopping in commercial chains.[17] India is one of the many developing countries considering such initiatives. But for such initiatives to succeed, national governments have to play a proactive role in setting food safety standards, and in close partnership with the private sector, enforce them. The latter, of course, is a major challenge given misleading labels and complex food chains across countries.

So the objective of influencing food choices is a daunting one because of the complex interplay of food prices and food preferences, and more so as evolution of food preferences is not well understood.[18] The state has to play a proactive role in combination with the private sector in ensuring that consumers make healthy food choices. As argued, it is far from obvious whether and how the media could promote healthy food choices when their vested interests lie elsewhere. We do not rule out effective regulation, but it would be naïve to be optimistic.

MIX OF PREVENTION AND TREATMENT OF NCDs

As noted in Chapter 7, foetal and childhood undernutrition is recognized as a long-term risk factor in the development of chronic diseases such as heart diseases, diabetes, hypertension, and stroke. India is struggling with undernutrition as many adults were exposed to undernutrition when they were young, creating a large pool of those at elevated risks (World Bank 2011).

Healthy ageing is thus crucial for tackling NCDs. Lessons learnt from developed countries point to many opportunities for their prevention and control. These relate to changes in risk levels within the population, and through primary care for NCDs.

A basic issue is whether governments should focus more on prevention of NCDs or on treating those already affected. In parallel, whether government should focus more on populations or on individuals? There have been advances in both knowledge of risk factors and their roles in causing NCDs, and effective treatments to lower the risk of complications. While generalizations are risky—primarily because cost-effectiveness analyses of specific interventions are few and far between—a few important insights are discussed.

Briefly, population-based interventions include health education through the mass media (relating to blood pressure, cholesterol concentration, and body mass), and agreements/legislation on salt content and step-wise decreases in salt content of processed foods, and restrictions on tobacco and alcohol consumption. Individualized health-service interventions include, for example, detection and treatment of people with high concentrations of cholesterol, and treatment of people with high systolic blood pressure.

In an important contribution, Murray *et al.* (2003) suggest that the optimum strategy is a combination of the population-based and individualized interventions. But if resources are scarce, as in India, the population-based interventions have higher priority.

As the evidence is sparse and confined to a few NCDs in specific countries, it is cited for illustrative purposes (World Bank 2011). If the tobacco and salt interventions are implemented jointly, it is estimated that 13.8 million deaths could be averted, at a cost of less than $0.40 per person a year in low-income and middle-income countries. In terms of absolute population numbers, the biggest gains are in countries with the largest population such as China and India.

Substitution of predominantly saturated palm oil with soyabean oil, high in unsaturated fatty acids, reduced cholesterol concentration by 14 per cent over a period of five years. Reduction in subsidies for butter reduced substantially mortality from cardiovascular disease (CVD).

Moving from a population-based level to a more focused, higher-risk approach, a recent study (Ramachandran *et al.* 2006) demonstrates the effectiveness of lifestyle modification involving moderate, but consistent, physical activity and diet modification in helping to prevent diabetes even in Asian Indians, who are highly prone to developing diabetes. Another study by Prabhakaran *et al.* (2009) reports reduction in CVD risk factors and intermediate CVD outcomes in India.[19]

Turning to individualized interventions, there is some evidence that a multi-drug regimen for the prevention of CVD could avert 17.9 million deaths from it in a sample of twenty-three countries over a ten-year period. The average annual cost per person would range from $0.43 to $0.90 in low-income countries and from $0.54 to $2.93 in middle-income countries. In India, the annual financial cost would be about 4 per cent of the annual health budget (World Bank 2011).

An important lesson from the extant literature is that, since risk factors tend to cluster (obesity, hypertension, and diabetes can occur in a single person, for example), health policy should target multiple common risks.

POLICY INITIATIVES IN AND OPTIONS FOR INDIA

Let us now consider policy initiatives in and options for India.[20] Proposed allocations for NCD programmes in the 11th Five Year Plan show that all NCD Control Programmes accounted for 28 per cent and Communicable Disease Control Programmes for the remaining 72 per cent. As the NCD burden is projected to rise sharply, a shift in health budget allocation in favour of the former is appropriate.[21]

A major initiative is the National Programme for Prevention and Control of Cancer, Diabetes, Cardiovascular Diseases and Stroke (NPCDCS). This will be implemented through primary health care centres and aim at: (i) assessment of risk factors, early diagnosis, and appropriate disease management for high risk groups; and (ii) health promotion for the general population (PHFI 2011). It is expected to be integrated into the health care system eventually and expanded to cover the entire country in the 12th Five Year Plan.

The Integrated Disease Surveillance Project was launched in 2004, in response to lack of data and systematic monitoring of NCDs. Phase 1 surveys were confined to CVD risk factors in the population and it is necessary now to collate information on associated mortality, complications, and health expenditure.

Under a related initiative—a Sentinel Surveillance System of Cardiovascular Disease Risk Factors in the Indian Industrial Population—on a small scale, local health care personnel in the participating industries were trained. The industry setting was the target, agent, and resource over four years. A population-based approach of behaviour change was the key feature of this intervention. This was augmented by high-risk individual counselling and policy change/environment approaches. The results were impressive. Significant reductions in population risk factors—including weight, waist circumference, blood pressure, and cholesterol—were observed. The proportion of participants with a ten-year CVD event risk score decreased significantly, while the control group showed a significant elevation (PHFI 2011).[22]

Another potentially effective intervention is a rural diabetes prevention programme in Chunampet, Tamil Nadu, under which screening is free, but about 60 per cent patients pay for their treatment at subsidized cost, while those who cannot afford the cost are treated free. The mean glycated haemoglobin levels among those diagnosed with diabetes decreased (PHFI 2011).

A youth-centric non-government organization (NGO), *HRIDAY*, has been engaged in promoting healthy behaviour among school students. Experimentation with tobacco, regular use of tobacco, and offer of tobacco by peers were all significantly reduced in the schools which implemented the programme in comparison with control or delayed intervention schools. This programme's success with promotion of healthy diets, physical activity, and environmental protection are now being replicated by other NGOs across India (PHFI 2011).

Some priorities in addressing the rising burden of NCDs are outlined below, which are essentially suggestive (PHFI 2011; World Bank 2011).

As we noted, there is a paucity of nationally representative and standardized data for most NCD risk factors and disease in India. The surveillance system is evolving and needs to be strengthened. A related concern is limited understanding of social, financial, behavioural, and organizational barriers that impede delivery of high quality NCD health care services. As the major NCDs have shared risks which present multiple opportunities for prevention and control, an overarching policy, linking actions in different sectors (health, non-health), is imperative. Different ministries such as health, rural development, finance, excise and taxes, education, agriculture, civil supplies, food processing, women and child development, among others, must coordinate their policies towards this goal. In addition, participation of civil society organizations, private health sector, media, and donor organizations is equally important for design and implementation of policies. The private sector has the potential for promoting healthy diets and physical activity, limiting levels of saturated fats, trans-fatty acids, sugars, and salts, and increasing availability of healthy and nutritious food choices. But whether these lofty goals will translate into a comprehensive policy for prevention and control of NCDs requires a vision and incentive compatible structures. For example, not just taxes and subsidies, but also effective mobilization and regulation of various stakeholders are needed.

Recalling the need for greater balance between population-based and individualized interventions, the verdict must be that it remains a distant and vague dream.

To conclude, our analysis covered a large ground in resolving the nutrition puzzle, dietary diversification, child malnutrition, PNT, prevalence of NCDs and their growing burden, and fragmented health policies. What is lacking is a vision that encompasses these concerns and a coordinated strategy that defines the roles of various stakeholders—the state, market, and communities—in the design and implementation of comprehensive policies towards mitigation of hunger, malnutrition, poverty, and vulnerability to disease.

NOTES

1. This curve denotes a relationship between calorie intake and income proxied by expenditure.
2. Note that these are distinct categories, but with some overlap. Hence, fast food is subsumed to include others for expositional convenience.
3. The Eurozone crisis refers to the current situation in large parts of Europe where several countries have accumulated huge private and public sector debts, and are in deep recession with no clear way out of it.

4. Comparison of NFHS-2 and NFHS-3 shows reductions in stunting and underweight rates while wasting rates increased.
5. This draws upon Gaiha and Kulkarni (2005), Gaiha *et al.* (2011), and Imai *et al.* (2012). The last is the most comprehensive analysis as it is based on two nationwide surveys conducted by the NCAER and three rounds of the NFHS (1, 2, and 3). Interestingly, some of the key findings are similar.
6. But these effects vary with the indicator and period(s) covered. For details, see Chapter 7 and Imai *et al.* (2012).
7. Several factors are associated with intra-uterine growth retardation (IUGR) and consequent low birth weight. These include maternal anemia and undernutrition, low age at marriage, short inter-pregnancy interval, and infections (Mendelson and Chaudhuri 2009). For a more recent review of evidence, see Kulkarni *et al.* (2013).
8. For an elaboration, see Imai and Sato (2010).
9. In fact, Ackerson and Subramanian (2008) report that preventing domestic violence could be as effective as the pharmaceutical approach of administering intestinal anthelmintic drugs.
10. For a cogently argued view focusing on women's property rights, see Panda and Agarwal (2005). For a more recent review focusing on the effects of violence against women and reproductive coercion, see WHO (2013), and Kulkarni *et al.* (2013).
11. Another study (Kandpal 2011), however, offers a more optimistic assessment on some criteria. Results show that ICDS increases height-for-age scores. As the average effects may mask variations in effectiveness, it is confirmed that ICDS also significantly improves height-for-age scores for the worst-off children.
12. For a clear and persuasive exposition, see Venu (2011). His estimate of foodgrain requirement is over 70 million tonnes—compared with the official claim that it should not exceed 60 million tonnes—to cover 75 per cent of the rural population and 50 per cent of the urban population.
13. Taxation of tobacco and alcohol is known to reduce their consumption significantly, and thus reduce the risks of NCDs—especially CVD (World Bank 2011).
14. Examining the portfolios of Coca Cola Company and PepsiCo, Popkin *et al.* (2012) report that while both total calories per capita and calories per ounce decreased in USA, the opposite was true in the developing markets of Brazil and China. Total calories per capita rose sharply in China and moderately in Brazil (Popkin *et al.* 2012).
15. As it turns out, the more important priority now is that safe and hygienically prepared meals are served.

16. Empirical evidence on the effectiveness of nutrition labeling, however, differs. A recent study conducted on parents of children aged 3–6 years shows that parents who were offered the nutritional menu card ordered food of lesser calorie. Another study, however, found no effect of provision of nutritional value on food ordering behaviour of adolescents (Kaushik *et al.* 2011).
17. Buckley's (2013) exposè of rat meat sold as mutton in China is shocking and stunning. In a show of bravado, the Ministry of Public Security announced '...that the police had caught a gang of traders in eastern China who bought rat, fox, and mink flesh and sold it as mutton. But that and other cases of meat smuggling, faking, and adulteration featured in Chinese newspapers and websites ... were unlikely to instil confidence in consumers already queasy over many reports about meat, fruit, and vegetables laden with disease, toxins, banned dyes, and preservatives. Firms based in developed countries are often just as guilty. A report in *The Economist* (2013), for example, drew attention to a New Zealand dairy firm, Fonterra, that found clostridium, a bacterium linked to botulism, in several batches of whey concentrate made in New Zealand and exported for use as an ingredient in infant milk powder. The contamination was traced to a dirty pipe. The tainted ingredient had been shipped to many countries. Another report in *The Economist* (February 2013) revealed that European food manufacturers—Tesco, a British supermarket, Aldi, a German discounter, and Findus, a frozen-food manufacturer—inadvertently sold horse meat as beef in burgers and lasagne. Horsemeat is not dangerous. Italian gourmets adore thin slices of *prosciutto di cavallo*. But if a product says 'beef' on the label, it should be that. Convoluted supply chains with expensive testing of food quality were the culprits, as the ground-up horse that found its way into the own-label lasagne of Findus and Aldi was apparently slaughtered in Romania.
18. In a deeply perceptive comment at the depths of the 'Great Depression', George Orwell wrote of the English working classes: 'The basis of their diet is white bread and margarine, corned beef, sugared tea, and potato—an appalling diet. Would it not be better if they spent more money on wholesome things like oranges and wholemeal bread?... Yes it would, but the point is, no human being would ever do such a thing... A millionaire may enjoy breakfasting off orange juice and Ryvita biscuits; an unemployed man does not... When you are underfed, harassed, bored, and miserable, you don't *want* to eat dull wholesome food. You want to eat something a little bit *tasty*.' (*The Economist*, March 2011).
19. Physical inactivity is a good predictor of CVD, type-2 diabetes, obesity, some cancers, and overall mortality. Men and women of all ages, socio-economic groups, and ethnicities are healthier if they achieve at least 150 min per week of moderate-intensity aerobic physical activity, such as brisk walking.

Even modest physical activity helps. Compared with inactive individuals, those who were active, but at levels less than recommended (150 min. per week), lived three years longer (Hallal *et al.* 2012).

20. Much of the evidence is drawn from PHFI (2011), using the framework delineated here—specifically, the mix of population-based policies and those relating to individual treatment.

21. It is estimated that the people with diabetes will increase from 40.9 million to 69.9 million by 2025; and obesity, which is associated with hypertension, CVD, diabetes, and some cancers, will affect 52.1 million by 2030. CVD is expected to be the main cause of death (37 per cent) by 2030 (World Bank 2011).

22. For other similar initiatives, see PHFI (2011) and World Bank (2011). At the state level, the Tamil Nadu Health System Project (TNHSP) is of particular interest, as it demonstrated that a primary health care approach, involving existing health services, has a high payoff in the detection and control of high blood pressure.

References

Ackerson, L.K. and S.V. Subramanian. 2008. 'Domestic Violence and Chronic Malnutrition Among Women and Children in India', *American Journal of Epidemiology*, 67(10): 1188–96.

Adkins, L.C. and R.C. Hill. 2008. *Using Stata for Principles of Econometrics*. Hoboken, NJ: John Wiley and Sons.

Afridi, F. 2010. 'Child Welfare Programs and Child Nutrition: Evidence from a Mandated School Meal Program', *Journal of Development Economics*, 92(2): 152–65.

Atkinson, A.B. 1987. 'On the Measurement of Poverty', *Econometrica*, 55(4): 749–64.

Bajpai, N., J. Sachs, and R.H. Dholakia. 2010. *Improving Access and Efficiency in Public Health Services: Mid-Term Evaluation of India's National Rural Health Mission*. New Delhi: Sage Publications.

Banerjee, A. and E. Duflo. 2011. *Poor Economics: Rethinking Poverty and the Ways to End It*. New Delhi: Random House India.

Banerjee, A. and A. Zucker. 2011. 'A First Look at the HUNGaMA Data', in *HUNGaMa Survey*.

Bardhan, P. 1984. *Land, Labour, and Poverty*. New York: Columbia University Press.

Barrett, C. 2002. 'Food Security and Food Assistance Programmes', in B. Gardner and G. Rausser (eds), *Handbook of Agricultural Economics*, pp. 2103–90. Amsterdam: Elsevier Science.

——— and P. Dorosh. 1996. 'Farmers' Welfare and Changing Food Prices: Non-parametric Evidence from Rice in Madagascar', *American Journal of Agricultural Economics*, 78(3): 656–69.

Behrman, J. and A. Deolalikar. 1987. 'Will Developing Country Nutrition Improve with Income? A Case Study for Rural South India', *Journal of Political Economy*, 95(3): 108–38.

Behrman, J. and A. Deolalikar. 1988. 'Health and Nutrition', in H. Chenery and T. N. Srinivasan (eds), *Handbook of Development Economics, Volume 1*, pp. 631–712. Amsterdam: North Holland, Elsevier.

———. 1989. 'Is Variety the Spice of Life? Implications for Calorie Intake', *The Review of Economics and Statistics*, 71(4): 666–72.

———. 1990. 'The Intrahousehold Demand for Nutrients in Rural South India: Individual Estimates, Fixed Estimates, and Permanent Income', *Journal of Human Resources*, 25(4): 665–97.

Bhalotra, S. 2004. 'Welfare Implications of Fiscal Reform: The Case of Food Subsidies in India', Chapter 11, in T. Addison and A. Roe (eds), *Fiscal Policy for Development: Poverty, Reconstruction, and Growth*, pp. 237–59. Houndmills, Basingstoke, Hampshire: Palgrave Macmillan.

Binswanger, H. and M. Rosenzweig. 1984. 'Contractual Arrangements, Employment and Wages in Rural Labour Markets: A Critical Review', in H. Binswanger and M. Rosenzweig (eds), *Contractual Arrangements Employment and Wages in Rural Labour Markets in Asia*, pp. 1–40. New Haven, Conn.: Yale University Press.

Bliss, C. and N. Stern. 1978a. 'Productivity, Wages and Nutrition: Part I: The Theory', *Journal of Development Economics*, 5(4): 331–62.

———. 1978b. 'Productivity, Wages, and Nutrition: Part II: Some Observations', *Journal of Development Economics*, 5(4): 363–98.

Bloom, D., D. Canning, and G. Fink. 2009. 'Disease and Development Revisited', *NBER Working Paper 15137*. Cambridge, MA.

Boerma, J.T., A.E. Sommerfelt, and G.T. Bicego. 1992. 'Child Anthropometry in Cross-Sectional Surveys in Developing Countries: An Assessment of the Survivor Bias', *American Journal of Epidemiology*, 135(4): 438–49.

Buckley, C. 2013. 'Rat Meat Sold as Lamb Highlights Fear in China', *The New York Times*, 3 May.

Chaudhury, N., J.S. Hammer, and A. Pokharel. 2008. 'First Things First: Infectious Disease, Child Mortality, and the Poor in India 1992–2005', mimeo, Washington DC: World Bank.

Dasgupta, P. 1993. *An Inquiry into Well-Being and Destitution*. Oxford: Clarendon Press.

———. 1997. 'Nutritional Status, the Capacity for Work, and Poverty Traps', *Journal of Econometrics*, 77(1): 5–37.

———. 2009. 'Poverty Traps: Exploring the Complexity of Causation', in J. von Braun, R.V. Hill, and R. Pandya-Lorch (eds), *The Poorest and the Hungry: Assessments, Analyses, and Actions*. Washington DC: IFPRI.

——— and D. Ray. 1986. 'Inequality as a Determinant of Malnutrition and Unemployment: Theory', *Economic Journal*, 96(384): 1011–34.

———. 1987. 'Inequality as a Determinant of Malnutrition and Unemployment: Policy', *The Economic Journal*, 97(385): 177–88.

Datt, G. and J. Olmsted. 2004. 'Induced Wage Effects of Changes in Food Prices in Egypt', *The Journal of Development Studies*, 40(4): 137–66.

Deaton, A. 1995. *The Analysis of Household Surveys: A Microeconomic Approach to Development Policy*. Baltimore: The Johns Hopkins University Press.

———. 2010. 'Price Indexes, Inequality and the Measurement of World Poverty', *American Economic Review*, 100(1): 5–34.

——— and A. Tarozzi. 2000. 'Prices and Poverty in India', mimeo, Princeton, NJ: Research Programme in Development Studies, Princeton University.

Deaton, A. and J. Dréze. 2009. 'Food and Nutrition in India: Facts and Interpretation', *Economic and Political Weekly*, 44(7): 42–65.

Deolalikar, A. 1988. 'Nutrition and Labour Productivity in Agriculture: Estimates for Rural South India', *Review of Economics and Statistics*, 70: 406–13.

———. 2010. 'The Middle Class in Asia: Emerging Trends and Patterns and their Implications', paper presented at a workshop on the *Asian Middle Class*, Asian Development Bank, 27–8 May.

Desai, S., A. Dubey, B. Joshi, M. Sen, A. Shariff, and R. Vanneman. 2010. *Human Development in India: Challenges for a Society in Transition*. New Delhi: Oxford University Press.

Dréze, J., and A. Goyal. 2003. 'Future of Mid-Day Meals', *Economic and Political Weekly*, 38(44): 4673–83.

The Economist. 2011. 'Nutrition Quality, not Quantity: Why Small Doses of Vitamins could make a Huge Difference to the World's Health?', 24 March.

———. 2013a. 'Food Safety: Spilt Milk: Now a Foreign Milk-Powder Producer has to say Sorry', 10 August.

———. 2013b. 'Horse Meat in the Food Chain is a Wake-Up Call, not a Calamity', 16 February.

———. 2013c. 'Indian Development: Beyond Bootstraps', a review of *An Uncertain Glory: India and its Contradictions*, by A. Sen and J. Dréze. 29 June. New York: Allen Lane.

Economist Intelligence Unit (EIU). 2012. *Global Food Security Index 2012*. London.

Eggleston, K., J. Oi, S. Rozelle, A. Sun, and X. Zhou. 2012. 'Aging Population and Poverty Require Stronger Investment in China's Rural Youth', Yale Global, 14 March.

FAO. 2012. 'The State of Food Insecurity in the World', Rome.

Food Safety and Standards Authority of India (FSSAI). 2012. 'Results-Framework Document for Food Safety and Standards Authority of India', New Delhi.

Gaiha, R. 1995. 'Does Agricultural Growth Matter in Poverty Reduction?', *Development and Change*, 26(2): 285–304.

———. 2003. 'Does the Right to Food Matter?', *Economic and Political Weekly*, 38(40): 4269–76.

Gaiha, R. and V.S. Kulkarni. 2005. 'Anthropometric Failure and Persistence of Poverty in Rural India', *International Review of Applied Economics*, 19(2): 179–97.

Gaiha, R., G. Thapa, K. Imai, and V.S. Kulkarni. 2007. 'Wages, Prices, and Anti-Poverty Interventions in India', Economics Discussion Paper Series–0723. Manchester: School of Social Sciences, University of Manchester.

———. 2008. 'Has Anything Changed? Deprivation, Disparity and Discrimination in Rural India', *Brown Journal of World Affairs*, 14(2): 113–25.

Gaiha, R., R. Jha, and V.S. Kulkarni. 2009. 'Who Has Most Say in Cooking?', ASARC Working Paper No. 19. Canberra: Australian National University.

———. 2010a. 'Obesity, Affluence, and Urbanization in India', Working Paper No. 2010/10, Australia South Asia Research Centre. Canberra: Australian National University.

———. 2010b. 'Prices, Expenditure, and Nutrition in India', Working Paper No. 2010/15, Australia South Asia Research Centre. Canberra: Australian National University.

Gaiha, R., V.S. Kulkarni, M.K. Pandey, and K. Imai. 2011. 'On Hunger and Child Mortality in India', *Journal of Asian and African Studies*, 47(1): 3–17.

Gaiha, R., R. Jha, and V.S. Kulkarni. 2012a. 'Demand for Nutrients in India: 1993 to 2004', *Applied Economics*, 45(14): 1869–86.

——— and N. Kaicker. 2012b. 'Diets, Nutrition and Poverty: The Indian Experience', in R.J. Herring (ed.), *Handbook of Food, Politics and Society* (forthcoming). New York: Oxford University Press.

Gaiha, R., R. Jha, and V.S. Kulkarni. 2013a. 'How Pervasive is Eating Out in India?', *Journal of Asian and African Studies*, 48(3): 370–86.

Gaiha, R., N. Kaicker, K.S. Imai, V.S. Kulkarni, and G. Thapa. 2013b. 'Has Dietary Transition Slowed in India? An Analysis based on the 50th, 61st, and 66th rounds of the National Sample Survey', Occasional Paper 16. Rome: Asia and the Pacific Division, IFAD.

Gopalan, C., B. Sastri, and S. Balasubramanian. 1971. *Nutritive Value of Indian Foods*. Hyderabad: National Institute of Nutrition, Indian Council of Medical Research.

Greene, W. 2003. *Econometric Analysis: Fifth Edition*. Upper Saddle River, NJ: Prentice Hall.

Gulati, A. and S. Fan (eds). 2007. *The Dragon and the Elephant: Agricultural and Rural Reforms in China and India*. Baltimore: Johns Hopkins University Press.

Gupta, A., J.P. Dadhich, and M.M. Faridi. 2010. 'Breastfeeding and Complementary Feeding as a Public Health Intervention for Child Survival in India', *The Indian Journal of Pediatrics*, 77(4): 413–18.

Hallal, P.C., A.E. Bauman, G.W. Heath, and H.W. Kohl. 2012. 'Physical Activity: More of the Same is Not Enough', *The Lancet*, 380(9838): 190–1.

Himanshu. 2007. 'Recent Trends in Poverty and Inequality: Some Preliminary Results', *Economic and Political Weekly*, 42(6): 497–508.

Himanshu and A. Sen. 2011. 'Why Not a Universal Food Security Legislation', *Economic and Political Weekly*, 46(12): 38–47.

Horton, S. and J. Ross. 2003. 'The Economics of Iron Deficiency', *Food Policy*, 28, 51–75.

HUNGaMA. 2011. *The HUNGaMA Survey Report, Citizens' Alliance Against Malnutrition*. Hyderabad: Naandi Foundation.

Imai, K. and T. Sato. 2010. 'Fertility, Parental Education, and Development in India: Evidence from National Household Survey Data', RIEB Discussion Paper series DP 2010–17. Kobe: Kobe University.

Imai, K., S.K. Annim, R. Gaiha, and V.S. Kulkarni. 2012. 'Does Women's Empowerment Reduce Prevalence of Stunted and Underweight Children in Rural India?', Economics Discussion Paper Series–1209. Manchester: School of Social Sciences, University of Manchester.

Indian Council of Medical Research (ICMR). 1990. *Nutrient Requirements and Recommended Dietary Allowances for Indians*. New Delhi: ICMR.

Institute of Applied Manpower Research (IAMR). 2011. *India Human Development Report: Towards Social Inclusion*. New Delhi: Oxford University Press.

Jensen, R.T. and N.H. Miller. 2011. 'A Revealed Preference Approach to Measuring Hunger and Undernutrition', mimeo.

Jha, R., R. Gaiha, and A. Sharma. 2009a. 'Calorie and Micronutrient and Poverty Nutrition Traps in Rural India', *World Development*, 37(5): 982–91.

———. 2009b. 'Modelling Variety in Consumption Expenditure on Food in India', *International Review of Applied Economics*, 23(4): 503–19.

Jha, R., S. Bhattacharya, and R. Gaiha. 2011. 'Social Safety Nets and Nutrient Deprivation: An Analysis of the National Rural Employment Guarantee Programme and the Public Distribution System in India', *Journal of Asian Economics*, 22(2): 189–201.

Jha, R., R. Gaiha, and M. Pandey, 2012. 'Body Mass Index, Participation, Duration of Work and earnings under NREGS: Evidence from Rajasthan', *Journal of Asian Economics*, 26(C): 14–30.

Jha, S. and B. Ramaswami. 2010. 'How Can Food Subsidies Work Better? Answers from India and the Philippines', Working Paper No 221, Asian Development Bank.

Kaicker, N., V.S. Kulkarni, and R. Gaiha. 2011. 'Dietary Transition in India: An Analysis Based on NSS Data for 1993 and 2004', paper presented at the World Congress of the International Economic Association, Beijing, 4–8 July.

Kandpal, E. 2010. 'Beyond Average Treatment Effects: Distribution of Child Nutrition Outcomes and Programme Placement in India's ICDS', *World Development*, 39(8): 1410–21.

Kapoor, C. 2009. 'Dealing with the Hidden Hunger of Our Children', *The Indian Express*, 6 April.

Kaushik, J.S., M. Narang, and A. Parakh. 2011. 'Fast Food Consumption in Children', *Indian Pediatrics*, 48(2): 97–101.

Khera, R. 2011. 'India's Public Distribution System: Utilization and Impact', *Journal of Development Studies*, 47(3): 1–23.

———. 2013. 'Mid-Day Meals: Looking Ahead', *Economic and Political Weekly*, 48(32): 12–14.

Kochar, A. 2005. 'Can Targeted Food Programmes Improve Nutrition? An Empirical Analysis of India's Public Distribution System', *Economic Development and Cultural Change*, 54(1): 203–35.

Kulkarni, V.S. and R. Gaiha. 2010. 'Dietary Transition in India', *India in Transition*. Philadelphia: CASI, University of Pennsylvania.

Kulkarni, V.S., M. Pandey, and R. Gaiha. 2013. 'MDGs and Gender Inequality', draft. Boston: Department of Global Health and Population, Harvard School of Public Health.

Kumar, R. and S.K. Ghosh. 2012. 'It Will Not Stop at Rs 60,000 Crore', *The Indian Express*, 15 February.

Lakdawala, D., T. Philipson, and J. Bhattacharya. 2005. 'Welfare Enhancing Technological Change and the Growth of Obesity', *The American Economic Review*, 95(2): 253–7.

Lanjouw, P. and M. Ravallion. 1995. 'Poverty and Household Size', *The Economic Journal*, 105(433): 1415–34.

Leibenstein, H. 1957. *Economic Backwardness and Economic Growth: Studies in the Theory of Economic Development*. New York: Wiley and Sons.

Mahal, A. and A. Karan. 2008. 'Adequacy of Dietary Intakes and Poverty in India: Trends in the 1990s', *Economics and Human Biology*, 6(1): 57–74.

Mahal, A., A. Karan, and M. Engelgau. 2010. *The Economic Implications of Non-Communicable Diseases for India*, HNP discussion paper. Washington DC: The International Bank for Reconstruction and Development/The World Bank.

Mazumdar, D. 1959. 'The Marginal Productivity Theory of Wages and Unemployment', *The Review of Economic Studies*, 26(3): 190–7.

Mendelson, S. and S. Chaudhuri. 2009. *Child Malnutrition in India: Why Does it Persist?* CINI.

Mirrlees, J. 1975. 'A Pure Theory of Underdeveloped Economies', in L. Reynolds (ed.), *Agriculture in Development Theory*, pp. 84–108. New Haven: Yale University Press.

Murray C.J.L., M. Ezzati, A.D. Lopez, A. Rodgers, and S. Vander Hoorn. 2003. 'Comparative Quantification of Health Risks: Conceptual Framework and Methodological Issues', *Population Health Metrics* (doi:10.1186/1478-

7954-1-1), available at http://www.pophealthmetrics.com/content/1/1/1 (accessed 8 March 2014).

Nandy, S. and J.J. Miranda. 2008. 'Overlooking Undernutrition? Using a Composite Index of Anthropometric Failure to Assess How Underweight Misses and Misleads the Assessment of Undernutrition in Young Children', *Social Science and Medicine*, 66(9): 1963–6.

Nandy, S., M. Irving, D. Gordon, S.V. Subramanian, and G.D. Smith. 2005. 'Poverty, Child Undernutrition and Morbidity: New Evidence', *Bulletin of the World Health Organization*, 83(3): 161–240.

OECD. 2011. *OECD Economic Surveys India*. Paris: OECD.

Osmani, S. 2000. 'Human Rights to Food, Health and Education', *Journal of Human Development*, 1(2): 273–98.

Panda, P. and B. Agarwal. 2005. 'Marital Violence, Human Development and Women's Property Status in India', *World Development*, 33(5): 823–50.

Pingali, P. 2007. 'Westernization of Asian Diets and the Transformation of Food Systems: Implications for Research and Policy', *Food Policy*, 32(3): 281–98.

Pitt, M. 1983. 'Food Preferences and Nutrition in Rural Bangladesh', *The Review of Economics and Statistics*, 65(1): 105–14.

——— and M. Rosenzweig. 1985. 'Health and Nutrient Consumption Across and Within Farm Households', *The Review of Economics and Statistics*, 67(2): 212–23.

———. 1986. 'Agricultural Prices, Food Consumption, and the Health and Productivity of Indonesian Farmers', in I. Singh, L. Squire, and J. Strauss (eds), *Agricultural Household Models: Extensions, Applications and Policy*, pp. 153–82. Baltimore: Johns Hopkins University Press.

Planning Commission. 2008. *Eleventh Five Year Plan*. New Delhi.

Popkin, B.M., L.S. Adair, and S.W. Ng. 2012. 'Global Nutrition Transition and the Pandemic of Obesity in Developing Countries', *Nutrition Reviews*, 70(1): 3–21.

Popkin, B.M., S. Horton, S. Kim, A. Mahal, and J. Shuigao. 2001. 'Trends in Diet, Nutritional Status, and Diet-Related Non-Communicable Diseases in China and India: The Economic Costs of the Nutrition Transition', *Nutrition Review*, 59(12): 379–90.

Prabhakaran, D., P. Jeemon, S. Goenka, R. Lakshamy, K.R. Thankappan, F. Ahmed, P.P. Joshi, B.V. Mohan, and K.S. Reddy. 2009. 'Impact of a Worksite Intervention Programme in Cardiovascular Risk Factors: A Demonstration Project in an Indian Industrial Population', *Journal of the American College of Cardiology*, 53(18): 1718–28.

Prasad, V., D. Sinha, and S. Sridhar. 2012. 'Falling Between Two Stools: Operational Inconsistencies between ICDS and NRHM in the Management of Severe Acute Malnutrition', *Indian Pediatrics*, 49(3): 181–5.

Public Health Foundation of India (PHFI). 2011. *Chronic Non-Communicable Diseases in India: Reversing the Tide*. New Delhi: PHFI.

Radhakrishna, R. and K. Subbarao, with S. Indrakant and C. Ravi (1997). 'India's Public Distribution: A National and International Perspective', World Bank Discussion Paper no. 380. Washington DC: The World Bank.

Ramachandran, A., C. Snehlata, S. Mary, B. Mukesh, A.D. Bhaskar, and V. Vijay. 2006. 'The Indian Diabetes Prevention Programme Shows that Lifestyle Modification and Metaformin Prevent Type 2 Diabetes in Asian Indian Subjects with Impaired Glucose Tolerance (IDPP-1)', *Diabetologia*, 49(2): 289–97.

Ramachandran, P. 2010. 'Nutrition and Child Survival in India', *The Indian Journal of Pediatrics*, 77(3): 301–5.

Ravallion, M. 1990. 'Rural Welfare Effects of Food Price Changes under Induced Wage Responses: Theory and Evidence for Bangladesh', *Oxford Economic Papers*, 42(3): 574–85.

Reddy, K.S., B. Shah, C. Varghese, and A. Ramadoss. 2005. 'Responding to the Threat of Chronic Diseases in India', *The Lancet*, 366: 1746–51.

Ruel, M.T., H. Alderman, and the Maternal and Child Nutrition Study Group. 2013. 'Nutrition–Sensitive Interventions and Programmes: How Can They Help to Accelerate Progress in Improving Maternal and Child Nutrition?', *The Lancet*, 382: 536–51.

Sah, R. and J. Stiglitz. 1987. 'Price Scissors and the Structure of the Economy', *Quarterly Journal of Economics*, 102: 109–34.

Sahn, D. and D.C. Stifel. 2002. 'Robust Comparisons of Malnutrition in Developing Countries', *American Journal of Agricultural Economics*, 84(3): 716–35.

Save the Children (SCR). 2012. *A Life Free from Hunger: Tackling Child Malnutrition*. London.

Sen, A. 1985. *Commodities and Capabilities*. Amsterdam: North Holland.

———. 1997. *On Economic Inequality* (expanded edition with a substantial annexe by J.E. Foster and A. Sen). Oxford: Clarendon Press.

———. 1999. *Development as Freedom*. New York: Knopf.

———. 2005. 'Description as Choice', *Oxford Economic Papers*, 32(3): 353–69.

——— and J. Dréze. 2013. *An Uncertain Glory: India and its Contradictions*. New York: Allan Lane.

Sen, A. and Himanshu. 2004. 'Poverty and Inequality in India – I', *Economic and Political Weekly*, 39(38): 4247–63.

Shetty, P.S. 2002. 'Nutrition Transition in India', *Public Health Nutrition*, 5(1A): 175–82.

Sinha, A. 2013. 'Food for Thought in a Mid-Day Meal Tragedy', *Business Standard*, 22 July.

Smith, G., S. Pellissery, S. Rajan, and S. Dubuc. 2007. *Indian Microdata Scoping Study: Final Report to the ESRC (2007)*. Available at http://www.esrc societytoday.ac.uk/ESRCInfoCentre/Images/Final%20Report%20-20India%20(PDF)_tcm6-19866.pdf (accessed 8 March 2014).

Smith, L., U. Ramakrishnan, A. Ndiaye, L. Haddad, and R. Matorell. 2003. 'The Importance of Women's Status for Child Nutrition in developing Countries', IFPRI Research Report 131. Washington DC: IFPRI.

Srinivasan, T.N. 1992. 'Undernutrition: Concepts, Measurements and Policy Implications', in S.R. Osmani (ed.), *Nutrition and Poverty*, pp. 97–120. Oxford: Clarendon Press.

Srinivasan, T.N. 1994. 'Destitution: A Discourse', *Journal of Economic Literature*, 32(4): 1842–55.

Stevens, G.A., M.M. Finucane, C.J. Paciorek, S.R. Flaxman, R.A. White, A.J. Donner, and M. Ezzati. 2012. 'Trends in Mild, Moderate, and Severe Stunting and Underweight, and Progress Towards MDG 1 in 141 Developing Countries: A Systematic Analysis of Population Representative Data', *The Lancet*, 380(9844): 824–34.

Strauss J. and D. Thomas. 1998. 'Health, Nutrition, and Economic Development', *Journal of Economic Literature*, 36(2): 766–817.

———. 1995. 'Human Resources: Empirical Modelling of Household and Family Decisions', in T.N. Srinivasan and J. Behrman (eds), *Handbook of Development Economics*, Volume III. Amsterdam: North Holland.

Subramanian, S. and A. Deaton. 1996. 'The Demand for Food and Calories', *Journal of Political Economy*, 104(1): 133–62.

Svedberg, P. 2000. *Poverty and Undernutrition: Theory, Measurement, and Policy*. Oxford: Oxford University Press.

———. 2004. 'Has the Relationship between Malnutrition and Income Changed?', comment on *Hunger And Malnutrition* by J. Behrman, H. Alderman and J. Hoddinott. Copenhagen: Copenhagen Consensus Opponent Note.

———. 2006. 'Declining Child Malnutrition: A Reassessment', *International Journal of Epidemiology*, 35(5): 1336–46.

———. 2007. 'Taking Action for the World's Poor and Hungry People', mimeo, Speaker Summary Note, Beijing, China, 17–19 October.

———. 2010. 'Estimates of Child Malnutrition in India', *Economic and Political Weekly*, 45(12): 14–18.

———. 2012. 'Reforming or Replacing the Public Distribution System with Cash Transfers', *Economic and Political Weekly*, 47(7): 53–62.

Swamy, A.V. 1997. 'A Simple Test of the Nutrition-Based Efficiency Wage Model', *Journal of Development Economics*, 53: 85–98.

Tarozzi, A. and A. Mahajan. 2007. 'Child Nutrition in India in the Nineties', *Economic Development and Cultural Change*, 55(3): 541–86.

Thomas, D. and J. Strauss. 1997. 'Health and Wages: Evidence on Men and Women in Urban Brazil', *Journal of Econometrics*, 77(1): 159–85.

Timmer, P.C. 1981. 'Is There "Curvature" in the Slutsky Matrix?', *The Review of Economics and Statistics*, 63(3): 395–402.

———. 1986. *Getting Prices Right: The Scope and Limits of Agricultural Price Policy*. Ithaca, NY: Cornell University Press.

———. 2008. 'Rural Changes Stimulate Rising Giants', *Science*, 321(5889): 642; review of *The Dragon and the Elephant: Agricultural and Rural Reforms in China and India*, by A. Gulati and S. Fan (eds), Baltimore: Johns Hopkins University Press.

———. 2009. 'Do Supermarkets Change the Food Policy Agenda', *World Development, Special Issue on Agrifood Industry Transformation, and Small Farmers in Developing Countries*, 37(11): 1812–19.

———. 2010. 'Reflections on Food Crises Past', *Food Policy*, 35: 1–11.

———, W.P. Falcon, and S.R. Pearson. 1983. *Food Policy Analysis*. Baltimore: Johns Hopkins University Press for the World Bank.

UNFPA. 2001. *The State of the World Population*. New York.

UNICEF. 2006. 'Progress for Children: A Report Card on Nutrition, Number 4'. Available at www.unicef.org/progressforchildren/2006n4/files/PFC4_EN_8X11.pdf (accessed 3 May 2013).

Venu, M.K. 2011. 'Securing Food Delivery', *The Indian Express*, 22 December.

Viswanathan, B. 2012. 'Counting Undernourished Children', *Economic and Political Weekly*, 47(20): 20–3.

Webb, P. and S.A. Block. 2004. 'Nutrition Information and Formal Schooling as Inputs to Child Nutrition', *Economic Development and Cultural Change*, 52(4): 801–20.

Weinberger, K. 2003. 'The Impact of Micronutrients on Labour Productivity: Evidence from Rural India', paper presented at the 25th International Conference of Agricultural Economists, Durban, South Africa, 16 August.

Weisell, R. and M.C. Dop. 2012. 'The Adult Male Equivalent Concept and its Application to Household Consumption and Expenditures Surveys (HCES)', *Food and Nutrition Bulletin*, 33(2): 157–62.

WHO. 2004. 'Appropriate Body-Mass Index for Asian Populations and Its Implications for Policy', *The Lancet*, 363(9403): 157–63.

———. 2006a. 'Obesity and Overweight', fact sheet no. 311.

———. 2006b. 'WHO Child Growth Standards Based on Length/Height, Weight and Age'. Available at www.ncbi.nlm.nih.gov/pubmed/16817681 (accessed 8 March 2014).

WHO. 2013. 'Global and Regional Estimates of Violence Against Women: Prevalence and Health Effects of Intimate Partner Violence and Non-Partner Sexual Violence'. Geneva.

Wooldridge, J.M. 2006. *Introductory Econometrics.* Mason, Ohio: Thomson South-Western.

World Bank. 2005. *Capitalising on the Demographic Transition: Tackling Non-Communicable Diseases in South Asia.* Washington DC: The World Bank.

———. 2006. *Repositioning Nutrition as Central to Development: A Strategy for Large Scale Action.* Washington DC: The World Bank.

———. 2011. *NCDs Policy Brief-India.* Washington DC: The World Bank.

Index

Editors and Contributors

Raghav Gaiha is Visiting Fellow in Economics, Australian National University (ANU). He was a professor of Public Policy, Faculty of Management Studies, University of Delhi. He also served as a visiting fellow/scholar at various institutions, including Harvard, MIT, Stanford, Yale, Penn, and University of Cambridge. His research interests lie in income distribution, agriculture, food prices, diets, malnutrition and disease, and rural public works and institutions. His recent publications include, *Battling Corruption: Has NREGA Reached India's Rural Poor?*, co-authored with Shylashri Shankar (OUP, 2013).

Raghbendra Jha, PhD (Columbia), FWIF, is Head, Arndt-Corden Department of Economics and Rajiv Gandhi Chair Professor of Economics, Executive Director of Australia South Asia Research Centre at the Australian National University (ANU) College of Asia and the Pacific. He has previously taught at Columbia University and Williams College in the US; Queen's University in Canada; University of Warwick in the UK; and Delhi School of Economics, Indian Institute of Management (IIM) Bangalore, and Indira Gandhi Institute of Development Research in India. His research and teaching areas include macroeconomics, public economics, and development economics. He has published almost 30 books and monographs with reputed publishers and more than 150 papers in scientific journals and other refereed outlets. His research has been funded by the Australian Research Council and Australian Agency for International Development (Australia), the MacArthur Foundation (US), Department for International Development (UK), IFAD (Rome), and IDRC and Shastri Indo-Canadian Institute (Canada). He has been a consultant for, among others, the World Bank, Citicorp, WIDER, UNRISD,

UNESCAP, ADB, IFAD, Future Foresight Project of the UK, the Reserve Bank of India, and the Government of India.

Nidhi Kaicker is an Assistant Professor at Ambedkar University, New Delhi. She holds an MBA degree from Faculty of Management Studies (FMS), University of Delhi. Her doctoral dissertation, completed at FMS, has been submitted to University of Delhi. She has published papers in Journal of Policy Modeling, and contributed chapters in R. Herring (ed.) *The Oxford Handbook of Food, Politics, and Society* (OUP New York, 2013). She has served as a consultant with IFAD, a UN agency. Her research interests include Financial Markets, Agriculture, Nutrition and Poverty and Financial Econometrics.

Vani S. Kulkarni is a postdoctoral Fellow in Sociology at Yale University, USA. She obtained a PhD with distinction at the University of Pennsylvania. She has held research fellowships and taught at Penn University, Harvard University, and Yale University. Her work lies at the intersection of racial-caste inequality, health, decentralized governance, gender, culture, and social theory. She has published in the ANNALS of the American Academy of Political and Social Science, *Journal of Asian and African Studies, Contemporary South Asia, Oxford Companion to Medical & Health Geography*, and an Encyclopaedia entry in Cultural Sociology of the Middle East, Asia, and Africa.

Manoj K. Pandey is a PhD candidate in Economics at the Australian National University (ANU), Australia. His prior affiliations include Australia South Asia Research Centre (ASARC) at the ANU, Institute of Economic Growth, and National Council for Applied Economic Research (NCAER), New Delhi. A researcher with strong background in applied econometrics and with a keen interest in interdisciplinary explorations, he has published in many journals of repute.

Anurag Sharma is a Senior Research Fellow in Faculty of Business and Economics, Monash University, Australia. His current research interests include Development Economics (poverty nutrition linkages and economics of education) and Health Economics (hospital choice modelling and impact of taxation strategies on consumption of soft drinks and alcohol).